Contributors

Audrey Knippa, MS, MPH, RN, CNE
Nursing Education Coordinator and
 Content Project Leader

Sheryl Sommer, PhD, MSN, RN
Director, Nursing Curriculum and
 Education Services

Brenda Ball, MEd, BSN, RN
Nursing Education Specialist

Lois Churchill, MN, RN
Nursing Education Specialist

Carrie B. Elkins, DHSc, MSN, PHCNS, BC
Nursing Education Specialist

Mary Jane Janowski, MA, BSN, RN
Nursing Resource Specialist

Karin Roberts, PhD, MSN, RN, CNE
Nursing Education Coordinator

Mendy G. Wright, DNP, MSN, RN
Nursing Education Specialist

Derek Prater, MS Journalism
Lead Product Developer and Editorial Project Leader

Erika A. Archer, BS Education, Foreign Language
Product Developer

Johanna Barnes, BA Journalism
Product Developer

Chris Crawford, BS Journalism
Product Developer

Hilary E. Groninger, BS Journalism
Product Developer

Megan E. Herre, BS Journalism
Product Developer

Amanda Lehman, BA English
Product Developer

Joanna Shindler, BA Journalism
Product Developer

Brant L. Stacy, BS Journalism, BA English
Product Developer

Consultants

Christina D. Brazier, MSN, RN

INTELLECTUAL PROPERTY NOTICE

IMPORTANT NOTICE TO THE READER

USER'S GUIDE

Welcome to the Assessment Technologies Institute® Nursing Leadership and Management Review Module Edition 5.0. The mission of ATI's Content Mastery Series® review modules is to provide user-friendly compendiums of nursing knowledge that will:

- Help you locate important information quickly.

- Assist in your remediation efforts.

- Provide exercises for applying your nursing knowledge.

- Facilitate your entry into the nursing profession as a newly licensed RN.

Organization

Chapters in this review module use a nursing concepts organizing framework, beginning with an overview describing the central concept and its relevance to nursing. Subordinate themes are covered in outline form to demonstrate relationships and present the information in a clear, succinct manner. Each chapter is divided into sections that group related concepts and contain their own overviews. These sections are included in the table of contents.

Application Exercises

Questions are provided at the end of each chapter so you can practice applying your knowledge. The Application Exercises include both NCLEX-style questions, such as multiple-choice and multiple-select items, and questions that ask you to apply your knowledge in other formats, such as short-answer and matching items. After the Application Exercises, an answer key is provided, along with rationales for the answers.

NCLEX® Connections

To prepare for the NCLEX-RN, it is important for you to understand how the content in this review module is connected to the NCLEX-RN test plan. You can find information on the detailed test plan at the National Council of State Boards of Nursing's Web site: https://www.ncsbn.org/. When reviewing content in this review module, regularly ask yourself, "How does this content fit into the test plan, and what types of questions related to this content should I expect?"

To help you in this process, we've included NCLEX Connections at the beginning of each chapter and with each question in the Application Exercises Answer Keys. The NCLEX Connections at the beginning of each chapter will point out areas of the detailed test plan that relate to the content within that chapter. The NCLEX Connections attached to the Application Exercises Answer Keys will demonstrate how each exercise fits within the detailed content outline.

These NCLEX Connections will help you understand how the detailed content outline is organized, starting with major client needs categories and subcategories and followed by related content areas and tasks. The major client needs categories are:

- Safe and Effective Care Environment

    ○ Management of Care

    ○ Safety and Infection Control

- Health Promotion and Maintenance

- Psychosocial Integrity

- Physiological Integrity
  - ○ Basic Care and Comfort
  - ○ Pharmacological and Parenteral Therapies
  - ○ Reduction of Risk Potential
  - ○ Physiological Adaptation

An NCLEX Connection might, for example, alert you that content within a chapter is related to:

- Management of Care
  - ○ Advance Directives
    - ■ Provide client with information about advance directives.

Icons

Icons are used throughout the review module to draw your attention to particular areas. Keep an eye out for these icons:

 This icon indicates an Overview, or introduction, to a particular subject matter. Descriptions and categories will typically be found in an Overview.

 This icon is used for the Application Exercises and the Application Exercises Answer Keys.

 This icon is used for NCLEX connections.

 This icon is used for gerontological content. When you see this icon, take note of information that is specific to aging or the care of older adult clients.

 This icon is used for content related to safety. When you see this icon, take note of safety concerns or steps that nurses can take to ensure client safety and a safe environment.

 This icon indicates that a media supplement, such as a graphic, an animation, or a video, is available. If you have an electronic copy of the review module, this icon will appear alongside clickable links to media supplements. If you have a hardcopy version of the review module, visit www.atitesting.com for details on how to access these features.

Feedback

ATI welcomes feedback regarding this review module. Please provide comments to: comments@atitesting.com.

Table of Contents

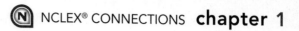

CHAPTER 1: MANAGING CLIENT CARE

- Leadership and Management
- Critical Thinking, Decision Making, Prioritization, and Time Management
- Assigning, Delegating, and Supervising
- Staff Education
- Performance Improvement
- Performance Appraisal, Peer Review, and Disciplinary Action
- Conflict Resolution
- Resource Management

NCLEX® CONNECTIONS

When reviewing the content in this chapter, keep in mind the relevant sections of the NCLEX® outline, in particular:

CLIENT NEEDS: MANAGEMENT OF CARE

Relevant topics/tasks include:
- Case Management
  - Plan safe, cost effective care for the client.
- Concepts of Management
  - Manage conflict among clients and health care staff.
- Delegation
  - Evaluate delegated tasks to ensure correct completion of activities.
- Establishing Priorities
  - Apply knowledge of pathophysiology when establishing priorities for interventions with multiple clients.
- Performance Improvement
  - Participate in performance improvement/quality assurance processes.
- Supervision
  - Evaluate the effectiveness of staff member's time management skills.

Chapter 1   Managing Client Care

 Overview

- Managing client care requires leadership and management skills and knowledge to effectively coordinate and carry out client care.

- To effectively manage client care, a nurse must develop knowledge and skills in several areas, including:

    o   Leadership and Management

    o   Critical Thinking, Decision Making, Prioritization, and Time Management

    o   Assigning, Delegating, and Supervising

    o   Staff Education

    o   Performance Improvement

    o   Performance Appraisal, Peer Review, and Disciplinary Action

    o   Conflict Resolution

    o   Resource Management

LEADERSHIP AND MANAGEMENT

 Overview

- Leadership and management are concepts that are integral to effective management and motivation of staff and clients. In their simplest terms:

    o   Management is getting work done through others.

    o   Leadership is the ability of an individual to influence the behavior of others.

- Effective managers usually possess good leadership skills; however, effective leaders are not always in a management position.

- Managers have formal positions of power and authority; leaders may have only the informal power afforded them by their peers.

- One cannot be a leader without followers.

Leadership

- Characteristics of Leaders

  - Initiative

  - Inspiration

  - Energy

  - Positive attitude

  - Communication skills

  - Respect

  - Problem-solving and critical-thinking skills

- Leaders have a combination of personality traits and leadership skills.

  - Great leaders were once thought to be born with skills that could not be acquired.

  - Contemporary leadership theory supports that leaders can develop the necessary skills.

- Leaders influence willing followers to move toward a goal.

  - Leaders have goals that may or may not reflect those of the organization.

- Transformational leaders empower followers to assume responsibility for a communal vision, and personal development is a secondary outcome.

- Transactional leaders focus on immediate problems, maintaining the status quo and using rewards to motivate followers.

Management

- Characteristics of Managers

  - Formal position of authority and power

  - Clinical expertise

  - Network

  - Coach

  - Decision maker

- Most managers can be categorized as authoritative, democratic, or laissez faire.

  - Authoritative

    - Makes decisions for the group.

    - Motivates by coercion.

    - Communication occurs down the chain of command.

    - Work output by staff is usually high – good for crisis situations and bureaucratic settings.

- o Democratic
  - Includes the group when decisions are made.
  - Motivates by supporting staff achievements.
  - Communication occurs up and down the chain of command.
  - Work output by staff is usually of good quality – good when cooperation and collaboration is necessary.
- o Laissez faire
  - Makes very few decisions and does little planning.
  - Motivation is largely the responsibility of individual staff members.
  - Communication occurs up and down the chain of command and between group members.
  - Work output is low unless an informal leader evolves from the group.
- o The use of any of these styles may be appropriate depending on the situation.
- The five major management functions are planning, organizing, staffing, directing, and controlling.
  - o Planning – The decisions regarding what needs to be done, how it will be done, and who is going to do it
  - o Organizing – The organizational structure that determines the lines of authority, channels of communication, and where decisions are made
  - o Staffing – The acquisition and management of adequate staff and staffing mix
  - o Directing – The leadership role assumed by a manager that influences and motivates staff to perform assigned roles
  - o Controlling – The evaluation of staff performance and evaluation of unit goals to ensure identified outcomes are being met

CRITICAL THINKING, DECISION MAKING, PRIORITIZATION, AND TIME MANAGEMENT

 Overview

- Critical thinking, decision making, prioritization, and time management are four skills necessary for nurses to be able to provide nursing care in an efficient and safe manner.
  - o Critical thinking is the mental process of analyzing or evaluating information.
  - o Decision making is the process by which a course of action is determined. The course of action may be in response to a problem or an issue.
  - o Prioritization is the organization of activities according to the order in which they should be done.
  - o Time management is the art of making the best use of time available to achieve specific tasks.

Critical Thinking

- Critical thinking reflects upon the meaning of statements, examines available data, and uses reason to make informed decisions.

- Critical thinking is necessary to reflect and evaluate from a broader scope of view.

- Sometimes one must think "outside the box" to come up with solutions that are best for clients, staff, and the organization.

- Critical thinking is more complex than decision making but is needed in order to make good decisions.

- Nurses must use good critical thinking skills when making decisions, prioritizing, and managing the care of clients.

Decision Making

- Decision making is a skill necessary for routine nursing activities but can also be applied to ethical issues.

- In decision making:

  - Objectives are defined.

  - Data are gathered.

  - Alternatives are determined.

  - Alternatives are evaluated in a logical and objective manner.

  - A decision is made and the choice is acted upon.

- Problem solving is a part of decision making.

  - Problem solving begins with a potential or actual threat or situation that needs or could benefit from an intervention.

  - The course of action may or may not resolve the problem on the first attempt.

  - The problem-solving model or the nursing process may provide a framework for solving client-related problems.

  - Steps included in the problem-solving model are:

    - The problem or issue is identified and defined.

    - Data are collected and analyzed in regard to the problem identified.

    - All possible solutions are identified and evaluated.

    - A solution is selected and implemented.

    - The results of the solution are evaluated.

Prioritization

- Nurses must continuously set and reset priorities in order to meet the needs of multiple clients and to maintain client safety.

- Priority setting requires that decisions be made regarding the order in which:

  o Clients are seen.

  o Assessments are completed.

  o Interventions are provided.

  o Steps in a client procedure are completed.

  o Components of client care are completed.

- Establishing priorities in nursing practice requires that these decisions be made based on evidence obtained:

  o During shift reports and other communications with members of the health care team

  o Through careful review of documents

  o By continuously and accurately collecting client data

PRIORITIZATION PRINCIPLES IN CLIENT CARE	
PRINCIPLE	EXAMPLES
Prioritize systemic before local ("life before limb").	• Prioritizing interventions for a client in shock over interventions for a client with a localized limb injury
Prioritize acute (less opportunity for physical adaptation) before chronic (greater opportunity for physical adaptation).	• Prioritizing the care of a client with a new injury/illness (e.g., mental confusion, chest pain) or an acute exacerbation of a previous illness over the care of a client with a long-term chronic illness
Prioritize actual problems before potential future problems.	• Prioritizing administration of medication to a client experiencing acute pain over ambulation of a client at risk for thrombophlebitis
Listen carefully to clients and don't assume.	• Recognizing that a postoperative client's report of pain could be due to pain in another location rather than expected surgical pain
Recognize and respond to trends versus transient findings.	• Recognizing a gradual deterioration in a client's level of consciousness and/or Glasgow Coma Scale score

NURSING LEADERSHIP AND MANAGEMENT

PRIORITIZATION PRINCIPLES IN CLIENT CARE	
PRINCIPLE	**EXAMPLES**
Recognize signs of medical emergencies and complications versus "expected client findings."	• Recognizing signs of increasing intracranial pressure in a client newly diagnosed with a stroke versus the clinical findings expected following a stroke
Apply clinical knowledge to procedural standards to determine the priority action.	• Recognizing that the timing of administration of antidiabetic and antimicrobial medications is more important than administration of some other medications

- Priority Setting Frameworks
  - Maslow's Hierarchy
    - The nurse should consider this hierarchy of human needs when prioritizing interventions. For example, the nurse should prioritize a client's:
      - Need for airway, oxygenation (or breathing), circulation, and potential for disability over need for shelter
      - Need for a safe and secure environment over a need for family support

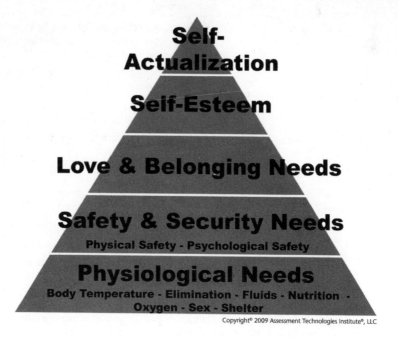

Self-Actualization

Self-Esteem

Love & Belonging Needs

Safety & Security Needs
Physical Safety - Psychological Safety

Physiological Needs
Body Temperature - Elimination - Fluids - Nutrition - Oxygen - Sex - Shelter

- ○ Airway Breathing Circulation (ABC) Framework
  - ■ The ABC framework identifies, in order, the three basic needs for sustaining life.
    - □ An open airway is necessary for breathing, so it is the highest priority.
    - □ Breathing is necessary for oxygenation of the blood to occur.
    - □ Circulation is necessary for oxygenated blood to reach the body's tissues.
  - ■ The severity of symptoms should also be considered when determining priorities. A severe circulation problem may take priority over a minor breathing problem.
  - ■ Some frameworks also include a "D" for disability, addressing the high priority given for prevention of disabilities.

PRIORITY	ASSESSMENT	INTERVENTIONS
First	Airway	• Identify an airway concern (obstruction, stridor). • Establish a patent airway if indicated. • Recognize that 3 to 5 min without oxygen causes irreversible brain damage secondary to cerebral anoxia.
Second	Breathing	• Assess the effectiveness of the client's breathing (apnea, depressed respiratory rate). • Intervene as appropriate (reposition, administer Narcan).
Third	Circulation	• Identify circulation concern (hypotension, dysrhythmia, inadequate cardiac output, compartment syndrome). • Institute appropriate actions to reverse or minimize circulatory alteration.
Fourth	Disability	• Assess for current or evolving disability (neurological deficits, stroke in evolution). • Implement action to slow down development of disability.

- ○ Safety/Risk Reduction
  - ■ Look first for a safety risk. For example, is there a finding that suggests a risk for airway obstruction, hypoxia, bleeding, infection, or injury?
  - ■ Next ask, "What's the risk to the client?" and "How significant is the risk compared to other posed risks?"
  - ■ Give priority to responding to whatever finding poses the greatest (or most imminent) risk to the client's physical well-being.
- ○ Assessment First
  - ■ Use the nursing process to gather pertinent information prior to making a decision regarding a plan of action. For example, determine if additional assessment information is needed prior to calling the primary care provider to ask for pain medication for a client.

     o   Survival Potential

- Use this framework for situations in which health resources are extremely limited (mass casualty, disaster triage).

- Give priority to clients who have a reasonable chance of survival with prompt intervention. Clients who have a limited likelihood of survival even with intense intervention are assigned the lowest priority.

     o   Least Restrictive

- Select interventions that maintain client safety while posing the least amount of restriction to the client. For example, if a client with a high fall risk index is getting out of bed without assistance, move the client closer to the nurses' work area rather than choosing to apply restraints.

Time Management

- Good time management:

  - Facilitates greater productivity.

  - Decreases work-related stress.

  - Helps ensure the provision of quality and appropriately prioritized client care.

  - Enhances satisfaction with care provided.

- Poor time management:

  - Impairs productivity.

  - Leads to feelings of being overwhelmed and stressed.

  - Increases omission of important tasks.

  - Creates dissatisfaction with care provided.

- Time management involves organizing care according to client care needs and priorities.

  - What must be done immediately (administration of analgesic or antiemetic, assessment of unstable client)?

  - What must be done by a specific time to ensure client safety, quality care, and compliance with facility policies and procedures (medication administration, vital signs, blood glucose monitoring)?

  - What must be done by the end of the shift (ambulation of the client, discharge and/or discharge teaching, dressing change)?

  - What can be delegated?

    - What can be done only by an RN?

    - What client care responsibilities can be delegated to other health care team members, such as licensed practical nurses (LPNs) and assistive personnel (AP)?

    - How can scheduled client care activities most efficiently be shared by these two groups of care providers?

- Time management involves using time-saving strategies and avoiding time wasters.

TIME SAVERS	TIME WASTERS
• Documenting nursing interventions as soon as possible after completion to facilitate accurate and thorough documentation	• Documenting at the end of the shift all client care provided and assessments done
• Grouping activities that are to be performed on the same client or are in close physical proximity to prevent unnecessary walking	• Making repeated trips to the supply room for equipment
• Estimating how long each activity will take and planning accordingly	• Providing care as opportunity arises regardless of other responsibilities
• Mentally envisioning the procedure to be performed and ensuring that all equipment has been gathered prior to entering the client's room	• Missing equipment when preparing to perform a procedure
• Taking time to plan care and taking priorities into consideration	• Failing to plan or managing by crisis
• Delegating activities to other staff when client care workload is beyond what can be handled by one nurse	• Being reluctant to delegate or underdelegating
• Enlisting the aid of other staff when a team approach would be more efficient than an individual approach	• Not asking for help when needed or trying to provide all client care independently
• Completing more difficult or strenuous tasks when energy level is high	• Procrastinating – delaying time-consuming, less desirable tasks until late in the shift
• Avoiding interruptions and graciously but assertively saying "no" to unreasonable or poorly timed requests for help	• Agreeing to help other team members when time is already compromised
• Setting a realistic standard for completion of care and level of performance within the constraints of assignment and resources	• Setting unrealistic standards for completion of care and level of performance within constraints of assignment and resources
• Completing one task before beginning another task	• Starting several tasks at once and not completing tasks before starting others
• Breaking large tasks into smaller tasks to make them more manageable	• Not addressing low level of skill competency, increasing time on task
• Using an organizational sheet to plan care	• Providing care without a written plan
• Using breaks to socialize with staff	• Socializing with staff during client care time

- Time management is a cyclic process.

    o Time initially spent developing a plan will save time later and help to avoid management by crisis.

    o Set goals and plan care based on established priorities and thoughtful utilization of resources.

NURSING LEADERSHIP AND MANAGEMENT

- ○ Complete one client care task before beginning the next, starting with the highest priority task.

- ○ Reprioritize remaining tasks based on continual reassessment of client care needs.

- ○ At the end of the day, perform a time analysis and determine if time was used wisely.

- Time Management and Teamwork

  - ○ Be cognizant of assistance needed by other health care team members.

  - ○ Offer to help when unexpected crises occur.

  - ○ Assist other team members with provision of care when experiencing a period of "down time."

- Time Management and Self-Care

  - ○ Take time for oneself.

  - ○ Schedule time for breaks and meals.

  - ○ Take physical and mental breaks from work/unit.

ASSIGNING, DELEGATING, AND SUPERVISING

 Overview

- Assigning is the process of transferring the authority, accountability, and responsibility of client care to another member of the health care team.

- Delegating is the process of transferring the authority and responsibility to another team member to complete a task, while retaining the accountability.

- Supervising is the process of directing, monitoring, and evaluating the performance of tasks by another member of the health care team. RNs are responsible for the supervision of client care tasks delegated to assistive personnel (AP) and licensed practical nurses (LPNs) – also known, respectively, as unlicensed assistive personnel (UAP) and licensed vocational nurses (LVNs).

  - ○ Licensed personnel are nurses who have completed a course of study and successfully passed either the NCLEX-PN or NCLEX-RN exam.

  - ○ Unlicensed personnel are specially trained to function in an assistive role to licensed nurses in client care activities.

    - These individuals may be nursing personnel, such as certified nursing assistants (CNAs) or certified medical assistants (CMAs), or they may be non-nursing personnel to whom nursing activities may be delegated, such as dialysis technicians, monitor technicians, and phlebotomists.

    - Some health care entities may differentiate between nurse and non-nurse assistive personnel by using the acronym NAP for nursing assistive personnel.

- RNs must delegate appropriately and supervise adequately to ensure that clients receive safe, quality care.

- Legal/ethical concerns must be considered when assigning and delegating.

  ○ The nurse leader should recognize limitations and use available information and resources to make the best possible decisions at the time.

  ○ Nurses must follow the ANA codes of standards in delegating and assigning tasks.

Assigning

- Assigning is done in a downward or lateral manner with regard to members of the health care team.

- Assignment Factors

  ○ Client factors

    ■ Condition of the client and level of care needed

    ■ Specific care needs (cardiac monitoring, mechanical ventilation)

    ■ Need for special precautions (isolation precautions, fall precautions, seizure precautions)

    ■ Procedures requiring a significant time commitment

  ○ Health care team factors

    ■ Knowledge and skill level of team members

    ■ Amount of supervision necessary

    ■ Staffing mix (RNs, LPNs, AP)

    ■ Nurse-to-client ratio

    ■ Experience with similar clients

    ■ Familiarity of staff member with unit

- When a nurse receives an inappropriate assignment, the following actions should be taken:

  ○ Bring the inappropriate assignment to the attention of the scheduling/charge nurse and negotiate a new assignment.

  ○ If no resolution is arrived at, take the concern up the chain of command.

  ○ If a satisfactory resolution is still not arrived at, an unsafe staffing complaint in the form of an Assignment Despite Objection (ADO) or Document of Practice Situation (DOPS) should be filed with the appropriate administrator.

  ○ Failure to accept the assignment without following the proper channels may be considered abandonment.

Delegating and Supervising

- A licensed nurse is responsible for providing clear directions when a task is initially delegated and for periodic reassessment and evaluation of the outcome of the task.

    ○ RNs may delegate to other RNs, LPNs, and AP.

        ■ RNs must be knowledgeable about the applicable state nurse practice act and regulations regarding the use of LPNs and AP.

        ■ RNs must delegate tasks so that they can complete higher level tasks that only RNs can perform. This allows more efficient use of all members of the health care team.

    ○ LPNs may delegate to other LPNs and AP.

- Delegation Factors

    ○ Nurses can only delegate tasks appropriate for the skill and education level of the health care provider who is receiving the assignment.

    ○ RNs cannot delegate the nursing process, client education, or tasks that require nursing judgment to LPNs or AP.

    ○ Task factors – Prior to delegating client care, the nurse should consider:

        ■ Predictability of outcome

            □ Will the completion of the task have a predictable outcome?

            □ Is it a routine treatment?

            □ Is it a new treatment?

        ■ Potential for harm

            □ Is there a chance that something negative may happen to the client (risk for bleeding, risk for aspiration)?

            □ Is the client unstable?

        ■ Complexity of care

            □ Are complex tasks required as a part of the client's care?

            □ Is the delegatee legally able to perform the task and does he have the skills necessary?

        ■ Need for problem solving and innovation

            □ Will a judgment need to be made while performing the task?

            □ Does it require nursing assessment skills?

        ■ Level of interaction with the client

            □ Is there a need to provide psychosocial support or education during the performance of the task?

- o Delegatee factors – Considerations for selection of an appropriate delegatee include:
    - Education, training, and experience
    - Knowledge and skill to perform the task
    - Level of critical thinking required to complete the task
    - Ability to communicate with others as it pertains to the task
    - Demonstrated competence
    - Agency policies and procedures and licensing legislation (state nurse practice acts)

EXAMPLES OF TASKS THAT CAN BE DELEGATED TO LPNs AND AP (PROVIDED AGENCY POLICY AND STATE PRACTICE GUIDELINES PERMIT)	
TO LPNs	TO AP
• Monitoring client findings (as input to the RN's ongoing assessment of the client) • Reinforcement of client teaching from a standard care plan • Tracheostomy care • Suctioning • Checking nasogastric tube patency • Administration of enteral feedings • Insertion of a urinary catheter • Medication administration (excluding intravenous medications in several states)	• Activities of daily living (ADLs) • Bathing • Grooming • Dressing • Toileting • Ambulating • Feeding (without swallowing precautions) • Positioning • Bed making • Specimen collection • Intake and output (I&O) • Vital signs (on stable clients)

- • Delegation and Supervision Guidelines
    - o Use professional judgment and critical thinking skills when delegating.
    - o Use the five rights of delegation to decide:
        - What tasks should be delegated (right task)
        - Under what circumstances (right circumstance)
        - To whom (right person)
        - What information should be communicated (right direction/communication)
        - How to supervise/evaluate (right supervision/evaluation)
    - o Right task
        - Identify what tasks are appropriate to delegate for each specific client.
            - □ A right task is repetitive, requires little supervision, and is relatively noninvasive for the client.
        - Delegate tasks to appropriate levels of team members (LPN, AP) based on standards of practice, legal and facility guidelines, and available resources.

RIGHT TASK	WRONG TASK
Delegate AP to assist a client who has pneumonia to use a bedpan.	Delegate AP to administer a nebulizer treatment to a client who has pneumonia.

- ○ Right circumstance
    - ■ Assess the health status and complexity of care required by the client.
    - ■ Match the complexity of care demands to the skill level of the health care team member.
    - ■ Consider the workload of the team member.

RIGHT CIRCUMSTANCE	WRONG CIRCUMSTANCE
Delegate AP to assist in obtaining vital signs from a stable postoperative client.	Delegate AP to assist in obtaining vital signs from a postoperative client who required naloxone (Narcan) for depressed respirations.

- ○ Right person
    - ■ Assess and verify the competency of the health care team member.
        - □ The task must be within the team member's scope of practice.
        - □ The team member must have the necessary competence/training.
    - ■ Continually review the performance of the team member and determine care competency.
    - ■ Assess team member performance based on standards and, when necessary, take steps to remediate a failure to meet standards.

RIGHT PERSON	WRONG PERSON
Delegate LPN to administer enteral feedings to a client who has a head injury.	Delegate AP to administer enteral feedings to a client who has a head injury.

- ○ Right direction/communication
    - ■ Communicate either in writing or orally:
        - □ Data that need to be collected
        - □ Method and timeline for reporting, including when to report concerns/assessment findings
        - □ Specific task(s) to be performed; client-specific instructions
        - □ Expected results, timelines, and expectations for follow-up communication

RIGHT DIRECTION/COMMUNICATION	WRONG DIRECTION/COMMUNICATION
Delegate AP the task of assisting the client in room 312 with a shower, to be completed by 0900.	Delegate AP the task of assisting the client in room 312 with morning hygiene.

- Right supervision/evaluation
  - The delegating nurse must:
    - Provide supervision, either directly or indirectly (assigning supervision to another licensed nurse).
    - Provide clear directions and understandable expectations of the task(s) to be performed (timeframes, what to report).
    - Monitor performance.
    - Provide feedback.
    - Intervene if necessary (unsafe clinical practice).
    - Evaluate the client and determine if client outcomes were met.
    - Evaluate client care tasks and identify needs for performance improvement activities and/or additional resources.

RIGHT SUPERVISION	WRONG SUPERVISION
After completing the admission assessment, an RN delegates to an AP the task of ambulating a client.	Prior to performing an admission assessment, an RN delegates to an AP the task of ambulating a client.

- Supervision occurs after delegation. A supervisor oversees a staff's performance of delegated activities and determines if:
  - Completion of tasks is on schedule.
  - Performance was at a satisfactory level.
  - Abnormal or unexpected findings were documented and reported.
  - Assistance is needed to complete assigned tasks in a timely manner.
  - Assignment should be re-evaluated and possibly changed.

STAFF EDUCATION

 Overview

- Staff education refers to the nurse's involvement in the orientation, socialization, education, and training of fellow health care workers to ensure the competence of all staff and to help them meet standards set forth by the facility and accrediting bodies. The process of staff education may also be referred to as staff development.

- The quality of client care provided is directly related to the education and level of competency of health care providers.

- The nurse leader has a responsibility in maintaining competent staff.

- Nurse leaders work with a unique, diverse workforce. Diversity should be respected and recognized.

Orientation

- Orientation helps newly licensed nurses translate the knowledge, skills, and attitudes learned in nursing school into practice.

- Orientation to the Institution

  ○ The newly licensed nurse is introduced to the philosophy, mission, and goals of the institution and department.

  ○ Policies and procedures that are based on institutional standards are reviewed.

  ○ Use of and access to the institution's computer system is a significant focus.

  ○ Safety and security protocols are emphasized in relation to the nurse's role.

- Orientation to the Unit

  ○ Classroom orientation usually moves onto the unit and is continued with an assigned preceptor.

  ○ Preceptors assist in orienting newly licensed nurses to a unit and supervising their performance and acquisition of skills.

  ○ Preceptors are usually assigned to newly licensed nurses for a limited amount of time.

  ○ Mentors may also serve as a newly licensed nurse's preceptor, but their relationship usually lasts longer and focuses more on assumption of the professional role and relationships, as well as socialization to practice.

Socialization

- Socialization is the process by which a person learns a new role and the values and culture of the group within which that role will be implemented.

  ○ Successful socialization helps new staff members fit in with already established staff on a client care unit.

  ○ Staff development educators and unit managers may begin this process during interviewing and orientation.

  ○ Nurse preceptors/mentors are frequently used to assist newly licensed nurses with this process on the clinical unit.

Education and Training

- Staff education, or staff development, is the process by which a staff member gains knowledge and skills. The goal of staff education is to ensure that staff have the most current knowledge and skills necessary to meet the needs of clients.

  ○ Staff education should be provided when new policies or procedures are put in place, when new equipment is introduced on a unit, and in relation to education needs identified by the unit manager or other staff members.

- o Staff education for an entire unit or department may be provided by peers, unit managers, and/or staff development educators, utilizing methods appropriate to the learning domain and staff learning styles.

- o Staff education needs by a particular staff member may be met on a one-on-one basis by the unit manager or charge nurse or the staff member's preceptor if one is in place.

- o "Just in time" training may be done by staff members who are working alongside or in a supervisory role to a colleague or subordinate who demonstrates an immediate need for training in relation to a client care task.

- o Staff education should also provide or encourage the attainment of a higher educational degree or certifications within a given field of expertise.

- • Educational programs should be provided using the following steps:

  - o Identify or respond to an identified educational need regarding a lack of knowledge or skill proficiency.

  - o Analyze the deficiency and develop learning objectives that address the need.

  - o Research resources available to address the learning objectives.

  - o Plan an educational program that addresses the learning objectives using the resources available.

  - o Implement the educational program at a time conducive to staff attendance. More than one session may be necessary or online modules may be made available for all staff.

  - o Use evaluative materials and observations to measure change in behavior secondary to learning objectives.

- • An increase in knowledge and competence is the goal of staff education.

  - o Competence is the ability of an employee to meet the requirements of a particular role at an established level of performance. Nurses will usually progress through several stages of proficiency as they gain experience in a particular area.

  - o Patricia Benner (1984) determined that nurses move through five stages of development, from novice to expert, in relation to level of competence. Level of competence is directly related to length of time in practice and exposure to clinical situations.

    - ■ Novice nurses have little clinical experience and approach client situations from a theoretical perspective relying on facts and established guidelines. Novice nurses are usually still in school but some new nurses may still function at this level.

    - ■ Advanced beginner nurses are able to practice independently on many tasks and can make some clinical judgments. Most new nurses function at this level.

    - ■ Competent, proficient, and expert nurses demonstrate increasing levels of skill proficiency and clinical judgment as they gain more experience, enhancing their ability to view situations holistically and process information more efficiently.

PERFORMANCE IMPROVEMENT

 Overview

- Performance improvement (quality improvement, quality control) is the process used to identify and resolve performance deficiencies. Performance improvement includes measuring performance against a set of predetermined standards. In health care these standards may be set by the specific facility and take into consideration accrediting and professional standards.

- Standards of care that are established should reflect optimal goals and be based on evidence.

- The performance improvement process focuses on assessment of outcomes and determines ways to improve the delivery of quality care. All levels of employees are involved in the performance improvement process.

- The Joint Commission's accreditation standards require institutions to show evidence of performance improvement in order to attain accreditation status.

Performance Improvement Process

- The performance improvement process begins with identification of standards and outcome indicators based on evidence.

  ○ Outcome, or clinical, indicators reflect desired client outcomes related to the standard under review.

  ○ Structure indicators reflect the setting in which care is being provided and the available human and material resources.

  ○ Process indicators reflect how client care is provided and are established by policies and procedures (clinical practice guidelines).

  ○ Benchmarks are goals that are set that determine at what level the outcome indicators should be met.

    ▪ While process indicators provide important information about how a procedure is being carried out, an outcome indicator measures whether that procedure is effective in meeting the desired benchmark. For example: the use of incentive spirometers in postoperative clients may be determined to be 92% (process indicator) but the rate of postoperative pneumonia may be determined to be 8% (outcome indicator). If the benchmark is set at 5%, the benchmark for that outcome indicator is not being met and the structure and process variables need to be analyzed to identify potential areas for improvement.

- Steps in the Performance Improvement Process

  ○ A standard is developed and approved by facility committee.

  ○ Standards are made available to employees by way of policies and procedures.

  ○ Quality issues are identified by staff, management, or risk management department.

- An interdisciplinary team is developed to review the issue.

- The current state of structure and process related to the issue is analyzed.

- Data collection methods are determined.

  - Quantitative methods are primarily used in the data collection process although client interview is also an option.

  - Audits can produce valuable quantitative data. There are several types of audits.

    - Types of Audits

      - Structure audits evaluate the influence of elements that exist separate from or outside of the client-staff interaction.

      - Process audits review how care was provided and assume a relationship exists between nurses and the quality of care provided.

      - Outcome audits determine what results, if any, occurred as a result of the nursing care provided.

    - Timing of Audits

      - Retrospective audits occur after the client receives care.

      - Concurrent audits occur while the client is receiving care.

      - Prospective audits predict how future client care will be affected by current level of services.

- Data is collected, analyzed, and compared with the established benchmark.

- If the benchmark is not met, possible influencing factors are determined. A root cause analysis may be done to critically assess all factors that influence the issue.

  - Root cause analyses focus on variables that surround the consequence of an action or occurrence.

  - Root cause analyses are commonly done for sentinel events (client death, client care resulting in serious physical injury) but may also be done as part of the performance improvement process.

  - A root cause analysis:

    - Investigates the consequence and possible causes.

    - Analyzes the possible causes and relationships that may exist.

    - Determines additional influences at each level of relationship.

    - Determines the root cause or causes.

- Potential solutions or corrective actions are analyzed and one is selected for implementation.

- Educational or corrective action is implemented.

- The issue is re-evaluated at a pre-established time to determine the efficacy of the solution or corrective action.

- The Nurse's Role in Performance Improvement

  o Serve as unit representative on committees developing policies and procedures. Use reliable resources for information (Centers for Disease Control and Prevention, professional journals, evidenced-based research).

  o Enhance knowledge and understanding of the facility's policies and procedures.

  o Provide client care consistent with these policies and procedures.

  o Document client care thoroughly and according to facility guidelines.

  o Participate in the collection of information/data related to staff's adherence to selected policy or procedure.

  o Assist with analysis of the information/data.

  o Compare results with the established benchmark.

  o Make a judgment about performance in regard to the findings.

  o Assist with provision of education or training necessary to improve the performance of staff.

  o Act as a role model by practicing in accordance with the established standard.

  o Assist with re-evaluation of staff performance by collection of information/data at a specified time.

PERFORMANCE APPRAISAL, PEER REVIEW, AND DISCIPLINARY ACTION

 Overview

- A performance appraisal is the process by which a supervisor evaluates an employee's performance in relation to the job description for that employee's position as well as other expectations the facility may have.

- Performance appraisals are done at regular intervals and may be more frequent for new employees.

- Performance expectations should be based on the standards set forth in a job description and written in objective terms.

- Performance appraisals allow nurses the opportunity to discuss personal goals with the unit manager as well as to receive feedback regarding level of performance. Performance appraisals can also be used as a motivational tool.

- Deficiencies identified during a performance appraisal or reported by coworkers may need to be addressed in a disciplinary manner.

Performance Appraisal and Peer Review

- A formal system for conducting performance appraisals should be in place and used consistently. Performance appraisal tools should reflect the staff member's job description and may be based on various types of scales or surveys.

- Various sources of data should be collected to ensure a nonbiased and thorough evaluation of an employee's performance.

  o Data should be collected over time and not just represent isolated incidents.

  o Actual observed behavior should be documented/used as evidence of satisfactory or unsatisfactory performance. These may be called anecdotal notes and are kept in the unit manager or equivalent position's files.

  o Peers can be a valuable source of data. Peer review is the evaluation of a colleague's practice by another peer. Peer review should:

    ▪ Begin with an orientation of staff to the peer review process, their professional responsibility in regard to promoting growth of colleagues, and the disposition of data collected.

    ▪ Focus on the peer's performance in relation to the job description or an appraisal tool that is based on institutional standards.

    ▪ Be shared with the peer and usually the manager.

    ▪ Be only part of the data used when completing a staff member's performance appraisal.

  o The employee should be given the opportunity to provide input into the evaluation.

- The performance appraisal review should be hosted by the unit manager in a private setting and held at a time conducive to the staff member's attendance. The unit manager should review the data with the staff member and provide the opportunity for feedback. Personal goals of the staff member should be discussed and documented, and avenues for attainment discussed. Staff members who do not agree with the unit manager's evaluation of their performance should have the opportunity to make written comments on the evaluation form and appeal the rating.

Disciplinary Action

- Deficiencies identified during a performance appraisal or the course of employment should be presented in writing, and corrective action should be based on institutional policy regarding disciplinary actions and/or termination of employment. Evidence regarding the deficiency must support such a claim.

- Some offenses such as mistreatment of a client or use of alcohol or drugs while working warrant immediate dismissal. Lesser infractions should follow a stepwise manner, giving the staff member the opportunity to correct unacceptable behavior.

  o First infraction – An informal reprimand or verbal warning should be the first course of action for minor offenses.

  o Second infraction – A formal reprimand or written warning should be the second course of action for selected, minor offenses.

  o Third infraction – Suspension from work or termination is usually the third or fourth course of action after the staff member has exceeded the established amount of time given to correct the behavior. Repeated offenses of the same infraction may precipitate additional disciplinary actions sooner than previously established.

- Staff members who witness an inappropriate action by a coworker should report the infraction up the chain of command. At the time of the infraction, this may be the charge nurse. The unit manager should also be notified, and written documentation by the manager may be placed in the staff member's permanent file.

CONFLICT RESOLUTION

 Overview

- Conflict is the result of opposing thoughts, ideas, feelings, perceptions, behaviors, values, opinions, or actions between individuals

- Conflict is an inevitable part of professional, social, and personal life and can have constructive or destructive results. Nurses must understand conflict and how to manage it.

- Problem-solving and negotiation strategies can often be used to prevent a problem from evolving into a conflict.

- Lack of conflict can create organizational stasis, while too much conflict can be demoralizing, produce anxiety, and contribute to burnout.

Categories of Conflict

- Intrapersonal conflict occurs within the person and may involve internal struggle related to contradictory values or wants.

  o Example: A nurse wants to move up on the career ladder but is finding that time with her family is subsequently compromised.

- Interpersonal conflict occurs between two or more people with differing values, goals, and/ or beliefs.

  o Interpersonal conflict in the health care setting involves disagreement among nurses, clients, family members, and within a health care team.

  o This is a significant issue in nursing, especially in relation to new nurses, who bring new personalities and perspectives to various health care settings.

  o Interpersonal conflict contributes to burnout and work-related stress.

    ▪ Example: A new nurse is given a client assignment that is heavier than those of other nurses, and when he asks for help, it is denied.

  o Intergroup conflict occurs between two or more groups of individuals, departments, or organizations and may be caused by a new policy or procedure, a change in leadership, or a change in organizational structure.

    ▪ Example: There is confusion as to whether it is the responsibility of the nursing unit or dietary department to pass meal trays.

Organizational Conflict

- Organizational conflict can disrupt working relationships and create a stressful atmosphere.

- If conflict exists to the level that productivity and quality of care are compromised, the unit manager must attempt to identify the origin of the conflict and attempt to resolve it.

- Common causes of organizational conflict include:

    o Ineffective communication

    o Unclear expectations of team members in their various roles

    o Poorly defined or actualized organizational structure

    o Conflicts of interest and variance in standards

    o Incompatibility of individuals

    o Management or staffing changes

    o Diversity related to age, gender, race, or ethnicity

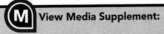 **View Media Supplement:**   Conflict Mediation (Video)

Conflict Resolution Strategies

- Problem Solving

    o Open communication among staff and between staff and clients can help defray the need for conflict resolution.

    o When potential sources of conflict exist, the use of open communication and problem-solving strategies can be effective tools to de-escalate the situation.

    o Steps of the problem-solving process that can be followed are:

        ▪ Identify the problem – State it in objective terms, minimizing emotional overlay.

        ▪ Discuss possible solutions – Brainstorming solutions as a group may stimulate new solutions to old problems. Encourage individuals to "think outside the box."

        ▪ Analyze identified solutions – The potential pros and cons of each possible solution should be discussed in an attempt to narrow down the number of viable solutions.

        ▪ Select a solution – Based on this analysis, select a solution for implementation.

        ▪ Implement the selected solution – A procedure and timeline for implementation should accompany the implementation of the selected solution.

        ▪ Evaluate the solution's ability to resolve the original problem – The outcomes surrounding the new solution should be evaluated according to the predetermined timeline. The solution should be given adequate time to become established as a new routine before it is evaluated. If the solution is deemed unsuccessful, the problem-solving process will need to be reinstituted and the problem discussed again.

- Negotiation

  ○ Negotiation is the process by which interested parties:

    ■ Resolve ongoing conflicts.

    ■ Agree on steps to take.

    ■ Bargain to protect individual or collective interests.

    ■ Pursue outcomes that benefit mutual interests.

  ○ Most nurses use negotiation on a daily basis.

  ○ Negotiation may involve the use of several conflict resolution strategies.

  ○ The focus is on a win-win solution or a win/lose-win/lose solution in which both parties win and lose a portion of their original objectives.

    ■ Each party agrees to give up something and the emphasis is on accommodating differences rather than similarities between parties.

    ■ For example, one nurse offers to care for Client A today if the other will care for Client B tomorrow.

CONFLICT RESOLUTION STRATEGIES	
STRATEGY	CHARACTERISTICS
• Avoiding/ Withdrawing	• Both parties know there is a conflict, but they refuse to face it or work toward a resolution. • May be appropriate for minor conflicts or when one party holds more power than the other party or if the issue may work itself out over time. • Since the conflict remains, it may surface again at a later date and escalate over time.
• Smoothing	• One party attempts to "smooth" another party by trying to satisfy the other party. • Often used to preserve or maintain a peaceful work environment. • The focus may be on what is agreed upon, leaving conflict largely unresolved. • This is usually a lose-lose solution.
• Competing/ Coercing	• One party pursues a desired solution at the expense of others. • Managers may use this when a quick or unpopular decision must be made. • The party who loses something may experience anger, aggravation, and a desire for retribution. • This is usually a win-lose solution.

CONFLICT RESOLUTION STRATEGIES	
STRATEGY	**CHARACTERISTICS**
• Cooperating/ Accommodating	• One party sacrifices something, allowing the other party to get what it wants. This is the opposite of competing. • The original problem may not actually be resolved. • The solution may contribute to future conflict. • This is a lose-win solution.
• Compromising/ Negotiating	• Each party gives up something. • To consider this a win/lose-win/lose solution, both parties must give up something equally important. If one party gives up more than the other, it can become a win-lose solution.

    ○   Consider the following example:

An experienced nurse on a urology unit arrives to work on the night shift. The unit manager immediately asks the nurse to float to a pediatrics unit because the hospital census is high and they are understaffed. The nurse has always maintained a positive attitude when asked to work on another medical-surgical unit but states she does not feel comfortable in the pediatric setting. The manager insists the nurse is the most qualified.

STRATEGY	CHARACTERISTICS
Avoiding/ Withdrawing	• The nurse basically cannot use these strategies due to the immediacy of the situation. The assignment cannot be simply avoided or smoothed over; it must be accepted or rejected.
Competing/Coercing	• If the nurse truly feels unqualified to work on the pediatric unit, then this approach may be appropriate – the nurse must win and the manager must lose. • Although risking termination by refusing the assignment, the nurse should take an assertive approach and inform the manager that children would be placed at risk.
Cooperating/ Accommodating	• If the nurse decides to accommodate the manager's request, then the children may be at risk for incompetent care. • Practice liability is another issue for consideration.
Compromising/ Negotiating	• This approach generally minimizes the losses for all involved while making certain each party gains something. • For example, the nurse might offer to work on another medical-surgical unit if someone from that unit feels comfortable in the pediatric environment. • Although each party is giving up something (the manager gives in to a different solution and the nurse still has to work on another unit), this sort of compromise can result in a win-win resolution.

Assertive Communication

- Use of assertive communication may be necessary during conflict negotiation.

- Assertive communication allows expression in direct, honest, and nonthreatening ways that do not infringe upon the rights of others.

- It is a communication style that acknowledges and deals with conflict, recognizes others as equals, and provides a direct statement of feelings.

- Elements of assertive communication include:

  ○ Selection of an appropriate location for the verbal exchange

  ○ Maintenance of eye contact

  ○ Establishing trust

  ○ Being sensitive to cultural needs

  ○ Speaking using "I" statements and including affective elements of the situation

  ○ Avoiding using "you" statements that can indicate blame

  ○ Stating concerns using open, honest, and direct statements

  ○ Conveying empathy

  ○ Focusing on the behavior or issue of conflict and avoiding personal attacks

  ○ Concluding with a statement that describes a fair solution

Grievances

- A grievance is a wrong perceived by an employee based on a feeling of unfair treatment that is considered grounds for a formal complaint.

- Grievances that cannot be satisfactorily resolved between the parties involved may need to be managed by a third party.

- All health care facilities have a formal grievance policy that should be followed when a conflict cannot be resolved.

- The steps of an institution's grievance procedure should be outlined in the grievance policy.

- Typical steps of the grievance process include:

  ○ Formal presentation of the complaint(s) using the proper chain of command

  ○ Formal hearing if the issue is not resolved at a lower level

  ○ Professional mediation if a solution is not reached during a formal hearing

RESOURCE MANAGEMENT

 Overview

- Resource management includes budgeting and resource allocation. Human, financial, and material resources must be considered.

  o Budgeting is usually the responsibility of the unit manager, but staff nurses may be asked to provide input.

  o Resource allocation is a responsibility of the unit manager as well as every practicing nurse.

  o Providing cost-effective client care should not compromise quality of care.

- Resources (supplies, equipment, personnel) are critical to accomplishing the goals and objectives of a health care facility, so it is essential for nurses to understand how to effectively manage resources.

Cost-Effective Resource Management

- Cost-effective resource allocation includes:

  o Using all levels of personnel to their fullest when making assignments.

  o Providing necessary equipment and properly charging clients.

  o Returning uncontaminated, unused equipment to the appropriate department for credit.

  o Using equipment properly to prevent wastage.

  o Providing training to staff unfamiliar with equipment.

  o Returning equipment (IV, kangaroo pumps) to the proper department (central service, central distribution) as soon as it is no longer needed. This action will prevent further cost to clients.

CHAPTER 1: MANAGING CLIENT CARE

 Application Exercises

1. A nurse receives a change-of-shift report at 0700 for an assigned caseload of clients. Number the following clients in the order in which they should be seen.

_____ A client who has been receiving a blood transfusion since 0400

_____ A client who has an every 4 hr PRN analgesic prescription and who last received pain medication at 0430

_____ A client who is going for a colonoscopy at 1130 and whose informed consent needs to be verified

_____ A client who needs rapid onset insulin before the 0800 trays arrive

_____ A client who is being discharged today and needs reinforcement of teaching regarding dressing changes

2. An older adult client who is on fall precautions is found lying on the floor of his hospital room. Which of the following actions is most appropriate for the nurse to take first?

   A. Call the client's primary care provider.

   B. Get staff to help you move the client back to bed.

   C. Inspect the client for injuries.

   D. Ask the client why he got out of bed without assistance.

3. A nurse receives the following change-of-shift report:

   28-year-old female admitted yesterday after surgery for a ruptured appendix
   Diagnosis: Peritonitis secondary to a ruptured appendix
   Vital signs: T 101° F, P 108/min, R 26/min, BP 148/78 mm Hg
   Oxygen 1 L/min per nasal cannula
   Pulse oximetry readings have decreased from 99% to 89% over the last 4 hr
   NPO except for ice chips
   Jackson Pratt drain: brown purulent fluid moderate amount
   D5½NS at 100 mL/hr via subclavian IV
   Morphine PCA, intermittent infusions of gentamicin (Gentacidin) and ceftriaxone (Rocephin) per prescribed schedule
   AM Lab Results:
      Hemoglobin 12.0 g/dL (preop 12.8 g/dL); Hematocrit 37% (preop 39%)
      Platelets 165,000/mm³ (preop 150,000/mm³)
      White blood cells 23,500/mm³ (preop 18,700/mm³)

   Based on the information provided in the change-of-shift report, the nurse should assign initial priority to which of the following reported client findings?

   A. Jackson Pratt drainage

   B. Heart rate

   C. Temperature

   D. Oxygen saturation level

4. A nurse is preparing to insert an intravenous catheter in a client who also needs to receive morphine sulfate 10 mg by intravenous bolus administration. Using time management principles, number the following steps in the order in which the nurse should perform them.

_____ Mentally envision the procedure when collecting supplies.

_____ Enter the room and perform hand hygiene.

_____ Draw up morphine sulfate and plan to administer immediately after IV is established.

_____ Explain the procedure and prepare the client.

_____ Notify staff members that she will be unavailable until the task is completed.

5. A charge nurse is preparing to make assignments for a busy surgical unit. Which of the following should the nurse consider when making shift assignments?

   A. The charge nurse should assume that since he is accountable for the care his clients receive, he is also responsible for carrying out that care.

   B. The charge nurse should delegate all possible client care to other levels of providers assigned to his clients (e.g., LPNs, AP).

   C. The charge nurse should collaborate with other levels of providers assigned to his clients and delegate care based on personal preference.

   D. The charge nurse should retain the client care activities that only an RN can perform and delegate other activities as appropriate.

6. Based on national guidelines rather than practice within any specific state, identify which team members can perform each of the following tasks. For some tasks, more than one team member can be designated.

TASK	AP	LPN	RN
Developing a teaching plan for a client newly diagnosed with diabetes mellitus			
Assessing a client admitted for surgery			
Collecting vital signs every 30 min for a client who is 1 hr post cardiac catheterization			
Calculating a client's intake and output			
Administering blood to a client			
Monitoring a client's condition during blood transfusions and intravenous administrations			
Providing oral and bathing hygiene to an immobilized client			
Initiating client referrals			
Dressing change of an uncomplicated wound			
Routine nasotracheal suctioning			
Receiving report from surgery nurse regarding a client to be admitted to a unit from the PACU			

TASK	AP	LPN	RN
Initiating a continuous IV infusion of dopamine with dosage titration based on hemodynamic measurements			
Administering subcutaneous insulin			
Assessing and documenting a client's decubitus ulcer			
Evaluating a client's advance directive status			
Providing written information regarding advance directives			
Initial feeding of a client who had a stroke and is at risk for aspiration			
Assisting a client with toileting			
Developing a plan of care for a client			
Administering an oral medication			
Assisting a client with ambulation			
Administering an IM pain medication			
Checking a client's feeding tube placement and patency			
Turning a client every 2 hr			
Calculating and monitoring TPN flow rate			
Administering morphine sulfate intravenously			

7. Toward the end of a shift, an LPN reports to an RN that a recently hired AP has not totaled clients' I&O for the past 12 hr. Which of the following actions should the RN take?

    A. Confront the AP about completing the intake and output measurements.

    B. Delegate this task to the LPN since the AP may not have been educated on this task.

    C. Ask the AP if assistance is needed to complete the I&O records.

    D. Notify the nurse manager to include this on the AP's evaluation.

8. As a part of orientation for new nurses, which of the following educational foci should be included? (Select all that apply.)

    _____ Skill proficiency

    _____ Assignment to a preceptor

    _____ Budgetary principles

    _____ Computerized charting

    _____ Socialization into unit culture

    _____ Facility policies and procedures

9. A new nurse witnesses an experienced nurse documenting an assessment of a patient-controlled analgesia (PCA) pump incorrectly on the computerized flow sheet. Which of the following should the new nurse do?

   A. Notify the charge nurse that the nurse has a staff development need.

   B. Leave a note for the unit manager that the nurse may have a learning need in regard to computerized charting.

   C. Bring to the nurse's attention that she is charting incorrectly and offer to demonstrate proper charting on the flow sheet.

   D. Question her own level of proficiency and seek out her preceptor for verification of correct procedure.

10. A nurse is participating in a performance improvement study of a procedure frequently performed on the unit. Which of the following will provide the most relevant information regarding the efficacy of the procedure?

    A. Frequency with which procedure is performed

    B. Client satisfaction with performance of procedure

    C. Incidence of complications related to procedure

    D. Accurate documentation of how procedure was performed

11. A nurse is hired to replace a staff member who has quit. After working on the unit for several weeks, the nurse notices that the unit manager does not intervene when there is conflict between team members, even when it escalates to a high level. Which of the following descriptions best describes the conflict resolution strategy the unit manager is employing?

    A. Avoiding/withdrawing

    B. Smoothing

    C. Cooperating/accommodating

    D. Negotiating

12. A nurse has just received a performance appraisal by the unit manager. Which of the following actions by the unit manager should be reported to the manager's supervisor?

    A. The evaluation was conducted in the unit manager's office.

    B. Data that was collected for the previous 12 months was presented.

    C. Verbal concerns provided by a staff member were incorporated into the data.

    D. The nurse was asked to review the performance appraisal tool and complete a self-evaluation.

CHAPTER 1: MANAGING CLIENT CARE

 Application Exercises Answer Key

1. A nurse receives a change-of-shift report at 0700 for an assigned caseload of clients. Number the following clients in the order in which they should be seen.

   1   A client who has been receiving a blood transfusion since 0400

   3   A client who has an every 4 hr PRN analgesic prescription and who last received pain medication at 0430

   4   A client who is going for a colonoscopy at 1130 and whose informed consent needs to be verified

   2   A client who needs rapid onset insulin before the 0800 trays arrive

   5   A client who is being discharged today and needs reinforcement of teaching regarding dressing changes

   1. The blood transfusion should not extend beyond 4 hr of infusion time. The nurse needs to check to make sure the client is tolerating the infusion well and that the transfusion is infusing correctly and is on time.

   2. The insulin will need to be administered before 0800.

   3. The nurse will need to evaluate for administration of an analgesic around 0830.

   4. The nurse should then verify that the informed consent is completed so as to allow sufficient time in case the nurse needs to take any action prior to the scheduled colonoscopy.

   5. The discharge teaching needs to be completed prior to discharge but is not as time sensitive as the other client interventions.

 NCLEX® Connection: Management of Care, Establishing Priorities

2. An older adult client who is on fall precautions is found lying on the floor of his hospital room. Which of the following actions is most appropriate for the nurse to take first?

   A. Call the client's primary care provider.

   B. Get staff to help you move the client back to bed.

   C. Inspect the client for injuries.

   D. Ask the client why he got out of bed without assistance.

   Using the assessment-first priority framework, it is most important to establish if the client has sustained any injuries and if emergency interventions are indicated. If emergency interventions are not indicated, the nurse should perform a focused assessment prior to calling the primary care provider. The client should not be moved without first determining the need for neck immobilization. Assessing the client's current condition is a priority rather than understanding the reason that the client attempted ambulation without assistance.

 NCLEX® Connection: Management of Care, Establishing Priorities

3. A nurse receives the following change-of-shift report:

> 28-year-old female admitted yesterday after surgery for a ruptured appendix
> Diagnosis: Peritonitis secondary to a ruptured appendix
> Vital signs: T 101° F, P 108/min, R 26/min, BP 148/78 mm Hg
> Oxygen 1 L/min per nasal cannula
> Pulse oximetry readings have decreased from 99% to 89% over the last 4 hr
> NPO except for ice chips
> Jackson Pratt drain: brown purulent fluid moderate amount
> D5½NS at 100 mL/hr via subclavian IV
> Morphine PCA, intermittent infusions of gentamicin (Gentacidin) and ceftriaxone (Rocephin) per prescribed schedule
> AM Lab Results:
>   Hemoglobin 12.0 g/dL (preop 12.8 g/dL); Hematocrit 37% (preop 39%)
>   Platelets 165,000/mm^3 (preop 150,000/mm^3)
>   White blood cells 23,500/mm^3 (preop 18,700/mm^3)

Based on the information provided in the change-of-shift report, the nurse should assign initial priority to which of the following reported client findings?

A. Jackson Pratt drainage

B. Heart rate

C. Temperature

D. Oxygen saturation level

According to the ABC priority setting framework, the client's oxygen saturation level should be assigned the highest priority.

 NCLEX® Connection: Management of Care, Establishing Priorities

4. A nurse is preparing to insert an intravenous catheter in a client who also needs to receive morphine sulfate 10 mg by intravenous bolus administration. Using time management principles, number the following steps in the order in which the nurse should perform them.

2	Mentally envision the procedure when collecting supplies.
4	Enter the room and perform hand hygiene.
3	Draw up morphine sulfate and plan to administer immediately after IV is established.
5	Explain the procedure and prepare the client.
1	Notify staff members that she will be unavailable until the task is completed.

1. Avoiding interruptions will help the nurse to stay focused and complete the task in a timely manner.

2. Mentally envisioning a procedure can help prevent omission of necessary equipment.

3. The morphine should be drawn up right before entering the room to prevent errors.

4. The next step is to go into the client's room and perform hand hygiene in preparation for completing the task.

5. The nurse has completed all preparation steps and is ready to start insertion of the IV.

 NCLEX® Connection: Management of Care, Establishing Priorities

5. A charge nurse is preparing to make assignments for a busy surgical unit. Which of the following should the nurse consider when making shift assignments?

A. The charge nurse should assume that since he is accountable for the care his clients receive, he is also responsible for carrying out that care.

B. The charge nurse should delegate all possible client care to other levels of providers assigned to his clients (e.g., LPNs, AP).

C. The charge nurse should collaborate with other levels of providers assigned to his clients and delegate care based on personal preference.

D. The charge nurse should retain the client care activities that only an RN can perform and delegate other activities as appropriate.

The nurse should begin the process of delegation by determining what he alone can do relative to his role as a professional nurse and team leader. While the nurse retains accountability for the care his clients receive, the nurse usually does not have the time to carry out all activities and should delegate selected responsibilities to other health care team members. However, the nurse may not want to delegate all possible care to other levels of providers, since this would significantly decrease client contact and informed care planning. After the nurse determines what should be delegated, these activities can then be distributed based on appropriate delegation guidelines.

 NCLEX® Connection: Management of Care, Delegation

6. Based on national guidelines rather than practice within any specific state, identify which team members can perform each of the following tasks. For some tasks, more than one team member can be designated.

TASK	AP	LPN	RN
Developing a teaching plan for a client newly diagnosed with diabetes mellitus			X
Assessing a client admitted for surgery			X
Collecting vital signs every 30 min for a client who is 1 hr post cardiac catheterization	X	X	X
Calculating a client's intake and output	X	X	X
Administering blood to a client			X
Monitoring a client's condition during blood transfusions and intravenous administrations		X	X
Providing oral and bathing hygiene to an immobilized client	X	X	X
Initiating client referrals			X
Dressing change of an uncomplicated wound		X	X
Routine nasotracheal suctioning		X	X
Receiving report from surgery nurse regarding a client to be admitted to a unit from the PACU			X
Initiating a continuous IV infusion of dopamine with dosage titration based on hemodynamic measurements			X
Administering subcutaneous insulin		X	X
Assessing and documenting a client's decubitus ulcer			X
Evaluating a client's advance directive status			X
Providing written information regarding advance directives		X	X
Initial feeding of a client who had a stroke and is at risk for aspiration			X
Assisting a client with toileting	X	X	X
Developing a plan of care for a client			X
Administering an oral medication		X	X
Assisting a client with ambulation	X	X	X
Administering an IM pain medication		X	X
Checking a client's feeding tube placement and patency		X	X
Turning a client every 2 hr	X	X	X
Calculating and monitoring TPN flow rate			X
Administering morphine sulfate intravenously			X

Rationale for RN-only tasks: RNs cannot delegate to LPNs or AP steps in the nursing process, client education, or tasks that require nursing judgment. In general, some input measures can be delegated (I&O, vital signs, reporting client observations), but not responsibility for the nursing process or clinical judgments.

Not all state practice acts allow for LPN performance of intravenous medication administration (intravenous bolus administration, blood administration, TPN).

Actions like titration of dopamine and feeding clients at risk for aspiration require nursing judgment.

 NCLEX® Connection: Management of Care, Delegation

7. Toward the end of a shift, an LPN reports to an RN that a recently hired AP has not totaled clients' I&O for the past 12 hr. Which of the following actions should the RN take?

    A. Confront the AP about completing the intake and output measurements.

    B. Delegate this task to the LPN since the AP may not have been educated on this task.

    C. Ask the AP if assistance is needed to complete the I&O records.

    D. Notify the nurse manager to include this on the AP's evaluation.

I&O measurements are routine AP tasks; however, the AP is new and may need some assistance. Making assumptions and negative evaluation without direct evidence should be avoided.

 NCLEX® Connection: Management of Care, Delegation

8. As a part of orientation for new nurses, which of the following educational foci should be included? (Select all that apply.)

X	**Skill proficiency**
X	**Assignment to a preceptor**
_____	Budgetary principles
X	**Computerized charting**
X	**Socialization into unit culture**
X	**Facility policies and procedures**

All of the above except budgetary principles need to be included in the orientation of new nurses. They need support in relation to transitioning to their first job, as well as becoming socialized into their new unit's culture. Budgetary principles are a higher-level administrative skill that is usually the responsibility of the unit manager.

 NCLEX® Connection: Management of Care, Continuity of Care

9. A new nurse witnesses an experienced nurse documenting an assessment of a patient-controlled analgesia (PCA) pump incorrectly on the computerized flow sheet. Which of the following should the new nurse do?

    A. Notify the charge nurse that the nurse has a staff development need.

    B. Leave a note for the unit manager that the nurse may have a learning need in regard to computerized charting.

    C. Bring to the nurse's attention that she is charting incorrectly and offer to demonstrate proper charting on the flow sheet.

    D. Question her own level of proficiency and seek out her preceptor for verification of correct procedure.

It is every nurse's responsibility to observe for and report or correct unsafe practices. Regardless of how experienced the nurse is, if the skill observed is within her purview of practice, she has the responsibility to attempt to correct and educate the other nurse in relation to proper charting. If the other nurse is not receptive to her interventions, then the new nurse should speak with the unit manager regarding her concerns.

 NCLEX® Connection: Management of Care, Performance Improvement

10. A nurse is participating in a performance improvement study of a procedure frequently performed on the unit. Which of the following will provide the most relevant information regarding the efficacy of the procedure?

    A. Frequency with which procedure is performed

    B. Client satisfaction with performance of procedure

    C. Incidence of complications related to procedure

    D. Accurate documentation of how procedure was performed

While all of the above are focused on some element of the performance improvement process, the primary focus of performance improvement is to determine if standards set by the institution are being met. The incidence of infections will indicate the quality of the outcomes and, subsequently, whether standards are being met in regard to the selected procedure.

 NCLEX® Connection: Management of Care, Performance Improvement

11. A nurse is hired to replace a staff member who has quit. After working on the unit for several weeks, the nurse notices that the unit manager does not intervene when there is conflict between team members, even when it escalates to a high level. Which of the following descriptions best describes the conflict resolution strategy the unit manager is employing?

    A. Avoiding/withdrawing

    B. Smoothing

    C. Cooperating/accommodating

    D. Negotiating

Environments that support a high level of conflict can be quite demoralizing and anxiety producing, which contributes to burnout. While it is possible that there could be open and honest communication and motivation for change on this unit, the likelihood is undermined by the excessive level of conflict being tolerated by management. The unit manager is not addressing conflict and is subsequently using the avoiding/withdrawing conflict resolution strategy.

 NCLEX® Connection: Management of Care, Concepts of Management

12. A nurse has just received a performance appraisal by the unit manager. Which of the following actions by the unit manager should be reported to the manager's supervisor?

    A. The evaluation was conducted in the unit manager's office.

    B. Data that was collected for the previous 12 months was presented.

    C. Verbal concerns provided by a staff member were incorporated into the data.

    D. The nurse was asked to review the performance appraisal tool and complete a self-evaluation.

All of the actions by the unit manager were acceptable practices regarding performance appraisal procedures except for incorporating concerns provided by another staff member into the evaluation data. The unit manager should only use data that has been observed and formally documented.

 NCLEX® Connection: Management of Care, Supervision

CHAPTER 2: COORDINATING CLIENT CARE

- Collaboration with the Interdisciplinary Team

- Principles of Case Management

- Continuity of Care: Consultations, Referrals, Transfers, and Discharge Planning

---

NCLEX® CONNECTIONS

When reviewing the content in this chapter, keep in mind the relevant sections of the NCLEX® outline, in particular:

CLIENT NEEDS: MANAGEMENT OF CARE

Relevant topics/tasks include:

- Case Management
  - Explore resources available to assist the client with achieving or maintaining independence.
- Collaboration with Interdisciplinary Team
  - Review the plan of care to ensure continuity across disciplines.
- Concepts of Management
  - Act as a liaison between the client and others.
- Consultation
  - Use clinical decision making/critical thinking in consultation situations.
- Continuity of Care
  - Maintain continuity of care between/among health care agencies.
- Referrals
  - Identify community resources for the client.

Chapter 2	Coordinating Client Care

 Overview

- One of the primary roles of nursing is the coordination and management of client care in collaboration with the health care team.

- In so doing, quality health care is provided as clients move through the health care system in a cost-effective and time-efficient manner.

- To effectively coordinate client care, a nurse must have an understanding of:

  o Collaboration With the Interdisciplinary Team

  o Principles of Case Management

  o Continuity of Care (including consultations, referrals, transfers, and discharge planning)

COLLABORATION WITH THE INTERDISCIPLINARY TEAM

 Overview

- An interdisciplinary team is a group of health care professionals from various disciplines.

- Collaboration involves discussion of client care issues in making health care decisions, especially for clients who have multiple problems. The specialized knowledge and skills of each discipline are used in the development of an interdisciplinary plan of care that addresses multiple problems. Nurses should recognize that the collaborative efforts of the interdisciplinary team allow the achievement of results that a team member would be incapable of accomplishing alone.

  o Nurse-primary care provider collaboration should be fostered to create a climate of mutual respect and collaborative practice.

  o Collaboration occurs among different levels of nurses and nurses with different areas of expertise.

  o Collaboration should also occur between the interdisciplinary team, the client, and the client's family/significant others when an interdisciplinary plan of care is being developed.

  o Collaboration is a form of conflict resolution that results in a win-win solution for both the client and health care team.

Nursing Role within the Interdisciplinary Team

- Qualities needed by the nurse for effective collaboration include:

  - Good communication skills

  - Assertiveness

  - Conflict negotiation skills

  - Decision making and critical thinking

- The nurse's role provides:

  - A holistic understanding of the client, the client's health care needs, and the health care system

  - The opportunity for care to be provided with continuity over time and across disciplines

  - Knowledge of a client's need for nursing care and its management

  - Information during rounds and interdisciplinary team meetings regarding the status of the client's health

  - An avenue for the initiation of a consultation related to a specific health care issue

  - A link to postdischarge resources that may need a referral

---

PRINCIPLES OF CASE MANAGEMENT

 Overview

- Case management is the coordination of care provided by an interdisciplinary team from the time a client starts receiving care until he or she is no longer receiving services.

- Case management focuses on managed care of the client through collaboration of the health care team in both inpatient and post-acute settings for insured individuals.

- A case manager collaborates with the interdisciplinary health care team during the assessment of a client's needs and subsequent care planning, and follows up by monitoring the achievement of desired client outcomes within established time parameters.

  - A case manager may be a nurse, social worker, or other designated health care professional.

    - A case manager's role and knowledge expectations are extensive; therefore, case managers are required to have advanced practice degrees or advanced training in this area.

  - A case manager nurse does not provide direct client care.

  - Case managers usually oversee a caseload of clients with similar disorders or treatment regimens.

  - Case managers in the community coordinate resources and services for clients whose care is based in a residential setting.

NURSING LEADERSHIP AND MANAGEMENT

- A critical or clinical pathway or care map may be used to support the implementation of clinical guidelines and protocols. These tools are usually based on cost and length of stay parameters mandated by prospective payment systems such as Medicare and insurance companies.

Nursing Role in Case Management

- The nurse's role in case management involves:

  - Coordinating care, particularly for clients with complex health care needs

  - Facilitating continuity of care

  - Improving efficiency of care and utilization of resources

  - Enhancing quality of care provided

  - Limiting unnecessary costs and lengthy stays

  - Advocating for the client and family

CONTINUITY OF CARE: CONSULTATIONS, REFERRALS, TRANSFERS, AND DISCHARGE PLANNING

 Overview

- Continuity of care refers to the consistency of care provided as clients move through the health care system. It enhances the quality of client care and facilitates the achievement of positive client outcomes.

- Continuity of care is desired as clients move from one:

  - Level of care to another, such as from the ICU to a medical unit

  - Facility to another, such as from an acute care facility to a skilled facility

  - Unit/department to another, such as from the PACU to the postsurgical unit

- Nurses are responsible for facilitating continuity of care and coordinating care through documentation, reporting, and collaboration.

- A formal, written plan of care enhances coordination of care between nurses, interdisciplinary team members, and primary care providers.

Nursing Role in Continuity of Care

- The nurse's role as coordinator of care includes:

  - Facilitating the continuity of care provided by members of the health care team

  - Acting as a representative of the client and as a liaison when collaborating with the primary care provider and other members of the health care team

    - When acting as a liaison, the nurse is usually serving as a client advocate.

- As the coordinator of care, the nurse is responsible for:

  o   Admission, transfer, discharge, and postdischarge orders

  o   Initiation, revision, and evaluation of the plan of care

  o   Reporting the client's status to other nurses and the primary care provider

  o   Coordinating the discharge plan

  o   Facilitating referrals and the utilization of community resources

Documentation and Communication

- Documentation to facilitate continuity of care includes:

  o   Graphic records that illustrate trending of assessment data such as vital signs

  o   Flow sheets that reflect routine care completed and other care-related data

  o   Nurses' notes that describe changes in client status or unusual circumstances

  o   Client care summaries that serve as quick references for client care information

  o   Nursing care plans that set the standard for care provided

    ■   Standardized nursing care plans provide a starting point for the nurse responsible for care plan development.

    ■   Standardized plans must be individualized to each client.

    ■   All documentation should reflect the plan of care.

- Communication and Continuity of Care

  o   Change-of-shift report

    ■   Performed with the nurse who is assuming responsibility for the client's care.

    ■   Describes the current health status of the client.

    ■   Informs the next shift of pertinent client care information.

    ■   Provides the oncoming nurse the opportunity to ask questions and clarify the plan of care.

    ■   Should be given in a private area, such as a conference room or at the bedside, to protect client confidentiality.

  o   Reports to the primary care provider

    ■   Assessment data integral to changes in client status

    ■   Recommendations for changes in the plan of care

    ■   Clarification of questionable orders

Consultations

- A consultant is a professional who provides expert advice in a particular area. A consultation is requested to help determine what treatment/services the client requires.

- Consultants provide expertise for clients who require a specific type of knowledge or service (a cardiologist for a client who had a myocardial infarction, a psychiatrist for a client whose risk for suicide must be assessed).

- Coordination of the consultant's recommendations with other health care providers' recommendations is necessary to protect the client from conflicting and potentially dangerous prescriptions.

- The nurse's role with regard to consultations is to:

  ○ Initiate the necessary consults or notify the primary care provider of the client's needs so the consult can be initiated.

  ○ Provide the consultant with all pertinent information about the problem (information from the client/family, the client's medical records).

  ○ Incorporate the consultant's recommendations into the client's plan of care.

  ○ Facilitate coordination of the consultant's recommendations with other health care providers' recommendations to protect the client from conflicting and potentially dangerous prescriptions.

Referrals

- A referral is a formal request for a special service by another care provider. It is made so that the client can access the care identified by the primary care provider or the consultant.

- The care may be provided in the inpatient setting (physical therapy, occupational therapy) or outside the facility (hospice care, home health aide).

- Clients being discharged from health care facilities to their home may still require nursing care.

- Discharge referrals are based on client needs in relation to actual and potential problems and may be facilitated with the assistance of social services, especially if there is a need for:

  ○ Specialized equipment (cane, walker, wheelchair, grab bars in bathroom)

  ○ Specialized therapists (physical, occupational, speech)

  ○ Care providers (home health nurse, hospice nurse, home health aide)

- Knowledge of community and online resources is necessary to appropriately link the client with needed services.

- The nurse's role with regard to referrals is to:

  ○ Begin discharge planning upon the client's admission.

  ○ Evaluate client/family competencies in relation to home care prior to discharge.

- o   Involve the client and family in care planning.

- o   Collaborate with other health care professionals to ensure all health care needs are met and necessary referrals are made.

- o   Complete referral forms to ensure proper reimbursement for prescribed services.

Transfers

- Clients may be transferred from one unit to another, one department to another, or one facility to another.

- Continuity of care must be maintained as the client moves from one setting to another.

- The nurse's role in regard to transfers is to provide a written and verbal report of the client's status and care needs including:

  - o   Client medical diagnosis and care providers

  - o   Client demographic information

  - o   Overview of client's health status, plan of care, and recent progress

  - o   Any alterations that may precipitate an immediate concern

  - o   Most recent set of vital signs and medications, including when a PRN was given

  - o   Notification of any assessments or client care that will be needed within the next few hours

  - o   Allergies

  - o   Diet and activity prescriptions

  - o   Presence of or need for special equipment or adaptive devices (oxygen, suction, wheelchair)

  - o   Advance directives and emergency code status

  - o   Family involvement in care and health care proxy, if applicable

View Media Supplement:

- Transfer Report (Image)
- Interfacility Transfer Form (Image)

Discharge Planning

- Discharge planning is an interdisciplinary process that is started by the nurse at admission.

  - o   The nurse conducts discharge planning with both the client and client's family for optimal results.

  - o   Discharge planning serves as a starting point for continuity of care. As client care needs are identified, measures can be taken to prepare for the provision of needed support.

  - o   The need for additional services such as home health, outpatient therapy, and respite care can be addressed before the client is discharged so the service is in place when the client arrives home.

- A client who leaves a facility without orders from the primary care provider is considered leaving "Against Medical Advice," or AMA. A client who is legally competent has the legal right to leave the facility at any time. A form, however, should be signed by the individual relinquishing responsibility for any complications that arise from discontinuing prescribed care.

- Discharge instructions should include:

  ○ Step-by-step instructions for procedures to be done at home

    ▪ Clients should be given the opportunity to provide a return demonstration of these procedures to validate learning.

  ○ Medication regimen instructions for home, including side effects and actions to take to minimize side effects.

  ○ Precautions to take when performing procedures or administering medications

  ○ Signs and symptoms of medication adverse effects or medical complications that should be reported to the provider

  ○ Names and numbers of health care providers and community services the client/family can contact

  ○ Plans for follow-up care and therapies

- The nurse's role with regard to discharge is to provide a written summary including:

  ○ Type of discharge (ordered by primary care provider, AMA)

  ○ Actual date and time of discharge, who accompanied the client, and how the client was transported (wheelchair to a private car, stretcher to an ambulance)

  ○ To where the client was discharged (home, long-term care facility)

  ○ A summary of the client's condition at discharge (steady gait, ambulating independently, blood glucose within normal limits)

  ○ A description of any unresolved difficulties and plans put in place for follow-up

  ○ Disposition of valuables, client's medications brought from home, and/or prescriptions

  ○ A copy of the client's discharge instructions

 View Media Supplement: Discharge Summary (Image)

CHAPTER 2: COORDINATING CLIENT CARE

 Application Exercises

1. When preparing the discharge of a client who has had a cerebrovascular accident and has a gastrostomy tube, the nurse should ensure that

    A. the client is independent in self-care.

    B. the family is able to give prescribed physical therapy in the home.

    C. instructions are provided for the enteral feedings that are to be done at home.

    D. prescribed medications are sent with the client.

2. Proper completion of discharge summaries when clients are transferred from one facility to another can facilitate _____ of care.

3. A nurse working on a rehabilitation unit attends an interdisciplinary team meeting. Her client, who experienced a cervical spinal cord injury in an automobile crash, will be discussed. Which of the following members of the interdisciplinary team should the nurse expect to be involved in developing the client's goals and plan of care? (Select all that apply.)

    _____ Speech therapist

    _____ Physical therapist

    _____ Occupational therapist

    _____ Physiatrist

    _____ Nurse

    _____ Vocational counselor

    _____ Psychologist

    _____ Respiratory therapist

4. Which of the following nursing actions support interdisciplinary collaboration? (Select all that apply.)

    _____ Open communication with team members

    _____ Acknowledgment of the knowledge and skill each discipline has to offer

    _____ Designation of a nurse who will serve as group facilitator

    _____ Invitation to the client and family to participate in the team meeting

    _____ Request for a referral

5. A nurse is preparing to discharge a client from an acute care facility to the skilled nursing unit of a long-term care facility. The client experienced a left-sided cardiovascular accident and has right-sided paralysis. She has been receiving physical, occupational, and speech therapy and has had problems with incontinence. What information is most important for the nurse to include in the discharge summary?

NURSING LEADERSHIP AND MANAGEMENT

6. A nurse is preparing to give a change-of-shift report regarding a client with a complex dressing change that is done every shift. The oncoming nurse has not cared for this client before. The oncoming nurse would like to see the client's dressing and asks if the nurse would provide report in the client's room. The client is in a semi-private room and has a roommate. Which of the following responses by the nurse preparing to leave is most appropriate?

    A. "Sure, just let me pick up the client's chart so I can give you report while we are in there and we can look at the procedure for changing the dressing, too."

    B. "Due to HIPAA regulations, we should not discuss client information in the room, so I will do my best to describe the dressing and how to change it during report in the conference room."

    C. "Let me give you report in the conference room first, and then we can visit the client and I will show you the dressing and how I have been changing it."

    D. "The orders for the dressing change are provided in detail in the client record. You should be able to change the dressing without difficulty if you follow them."

7. One of the names of the tool that is used by various members of the health care team to direct and focus a client's care is a _____.

CHAPTER 2: COORDINATING CLIENT CARE

 Application Exercises Answer Key

1. When preparing the discharge of a client who has had a cerebrovascular accident and has a gastrostomy tube, the nurse should ensure that

   A. the client is independent in self-care.

   B. the family is able to give prescribed physical therapy in the home.

   C. instructions are provided for the enteral feedings that are to be done at home.

   D. prescribed medications are sent with the client.

   Clients who still require nursing care, such as enteral feedings, may be discharged to home. It is the responsibility of the health care team to make sure they have been instructed on this care and that home care instructions are provided. Many clients who have had a cerebrovascular accident will continue to need assistance with their self-care, as well as physical therapy. Arrangements should be made for a visiting nurse, home health aide, and physical therapist to come to the home and continue this level of care. Medications should be obtained at a local pharmacy rather than the hospital or rehabilitation setting.

 NCLEX® Connection: Management of Care, Collaboration with Interdisciplinary Team

2. Proper completion of discharge summaries when clients are transferred from one facility to another can facilitate **continuity** of care.

 NCLEX® Connection: Management of Care, Continuity of Care

3. A nurse working on a rehabilitation unit attends an interdisciplinary team meeting. Her client, who experienced a cervical spinal cord injury in an automobile crash, will be discussed. Which of the following members of the interdisciplinary team should the nurse expect to be involved in developing the client's goals and plan of care? (Select all that apply.)

   _____ Speech therapist

   __X__ **Physical therapist**

   __X__ **Occupational therapist**

   __X__ **Physiatrist**

   __X__ **Nurse**

   __X__ **Vocational counselor**

   __X__ **Psychologist**

   __X__ **Respiratory therapist**

   Since cervical injuries cause extremely complex functional deficits, the interdisciplinary team will most likely consist of nurses, a medical doctor who specializes in rehabilitation or physiatrist, physical and occupational therapists, a respiratory therapist, a vocational counselor, and a psychologist. The speech therapist will not be needed because the client should not have any speech or swallowing difficulties.

 NCLEX® Connection: Management of Care, Collaboration with Interdisciplinary Team

4. Which of the following nursing actions support interdisciplinary collaboration? (Select all that apply.)

__X__ **Open communication with team members**

__X__ **Acknowledgment of the knowledge and skill each discipline has to offer**

_____ Designation of a nurse who will serve as group facilitator

__X__ **Invitation to the client and family to participate in the team meeting**

__X__ **Request for a referral**

Open communication and appreciation of the knowledge and skill of each discipline is critical for interdisciplinary decision making. Equal contributions by all members are necessary. When appropriate, the client and family should be included in the decision-making process. A nurse does not need to be the facilitator of an interdisciplinary team. The facilitator can be any member of the team involved in the client's care. A request for a referral invites another member of the interdisciplinary team to become involved in the client's care.

 NCLEX® Connection: Management of Care, Collaboration with Interdisciplinary Team

5. A nurse is preparing to discharge a client from an acute care facility to the skilled nursing unit of a long-term care facility. The client experienced a left-sided cardiovascular accident and has right-sided paralysis. She has been receiving physical, occupational, and speech therapy and has had problems with incontinence. What information is most important for the nurse to include in the discharge summary?

The discharge summary should include:

History of current illness, other coexisting illnesses

Current level of functional abilities, perhaps in the form of a functional assessment tool

Medical prescriptions from the primary care provider for medications and treatments

A summary of the physical, occupational, and speech therapy provided and current goals

Description of the bladder and bowel program instituted and the client or family education that has been provided

Status of the client upon discharge, mode of transportation, and who accompanied the client

 NCLEX® Connection: Management of Care, Continuity of Care

6. A nurse is preparing to give a change-of-shift report regarding a client with a complex dressing change that is done every shift. The oncoming nurse has not cared for this client before. The oncoming nurse would like to see the client's dressing and asks if the nurse would provide report in the client's room. The client is in a semi-private room and has a roommate. Which of the following responses by the nurse preparing to leave is most appropriate?

    A. "Sure, just let me pick up the client's chart so I can give you report while we are in there and we can look at the procedure for changing the dressing, too."

    B. "Due to HIPAA regulations, we should not discuss client information in the room, so I will do my best to describe the dressing and how to change it during report in the conference room."

    C. "Let me give you report in the conference room first, and then we can visit the client and I will show you the dressing and how I have been changing it."

    D. "The orders for the dressing change are provided in detail in the client record. You should be able to change the dressing without difficulty if you follow them."

Due to HIPAA regulations, nurses should not give report anywhere that the client's information could be overheard by individuals not involved in the client's care. Report should be given in a private location with a door, such as a conference room. Since the dressing change is complex, it is the responsibility of the nurse who is leaving to ensure that the oncoming nurse provides continuity of care by correctly performing the dressing change on her shift. This can be done after report by going into the room and quietly discussing only this facet of client care. Even though the orders for the dressing change are in the client record, the oncoming nurse has verbalized she is unsure of how to do it, so additional information and demonstration should be provided.

 NCLEX® Connection: Management of Care, Confidentiality/Information Security

7. One of the names of the tool that is used by various members of the health care team to direct and focus a client's care is a _____.

"critical pathway," "clinical pathway," or "care map"

 NCLEX® Connection: Management of Care, Collaboration with Interdisciplinary Team

CHAPTER 3: PROFESSIONAL RESPONSIBILITIES

- Client Rights
- Advocacy
- Informed Consent
- Advance Directives
- Confidentiality and Information Security
- Legal Practice
- Ethical Practice

NCLEX® CONNECTIONS

When reviewing the content in this chapter, keep in mind the relevant sections of the NCLEX® outline, in particular:

CLIENT NEEDS: MANAGEMENT OF CARE

Relevant topics/tasks include:
- Advance Directives
  - Integrate advance directives into the client's plan of care.
- Advocacy
  - Discuss identified treatment options with clients and respect their decisions.
- Client Rights
  - Educate clients and staff about client rights and responsibilities.
- Confidentiality/Information Security
  - Assess staff member and client understanding of confidentiality requirements.
- Ethical Practice
  - Recognize ethical dilemmas and take appropriate action.
- Information Technology
  - Use emerging technology in managing client health care.
- Informed Consent
  - Verify that the client comprehends and consents to care/procedures, including procedures requiring informed consent.
- Legal Rights and Responsibilities
  - Educate the client/staff on legal issues.

Chapter 3   Professional Responsibilities

 Overview

- Professional responsibilities are the obligations that nurses have to their clients.

- To meet their professional responsibilities, nurses must be knowledgeable in the following areas:

    o   Client Rights

    o   Advocacy

    o   Informed Consent

    o   Advance Directives

    o   Confidentiality and Information Security

    o   Legal Practice

    o   Ethical Practice

CLIENT RIGHTS

 Overview

- Client rights are the legal guarantees that clients have with regard to their health care.

    o   Clients using the services of a health care institution retain their rights as individuals and citizens of the United States. The American Hospital Association (AHA) identifies client rights in health care settings in "The Patient Care Partnership." For more information regarding this document, go to http://www.aha.org/.

    o   Residents in nursing facilities that participate in Medicare programs similarly retain "Resident Rights" under statutes that govern the operation of these facilities.

- Nurses are accountable for protecting the rights of clients. Situations that require particular attention include informed consent, refusal of treatment, advance directives, confidentiality, and information security.

Nursing Role in Client Rights

- Nurses must ensure that clients understand their rights, and nurses must also protect clients' rights during nursing care.

- Regardless of the client's age, the client's nursing needs, or the setting in which care is provided, the basic tenants are the same. Each client has the right to:

  ○ Be informed about all aspects of care and take an active role in the decision-making process.

  ○ Accept, refuse, or request modification to the plan of care.

  ○ Receive care that is delivered by competent individuals who treat the client with respect.

- Refusal of Treatment

  ○ The Patient Self-Determination Act (PSDA) stipulates that on admission to a health care facility all clients must be informed of their right to accept or refuse care. Competent adults have the right to refuse treatment, including the right to leave a health care facility without a discharge order from the primary care provider.

  ○ If the client refuses a treatment or procedure, the client is asked to sign a document indicating that he understands the risk involved with refusing the treatment or procedure and that he has chosen to refuse it.

  ○ When a client decides to leave the facility without a discharge order, the nurse notifies the primary care provider and discusses with the client the risks the client may face by leaving the facility prior to discharge.

  ○ The nurse carefully documents the information that was provided to the client and that notification of the primary care provider occurred. The client should be informed of the following:

    ▪ Possible complications that could occur without treatment.

    ▪ Possibility of permanent physical or mental impairment or disability.

    ▪ Possibility of other complications that could lead to death.

  ○ The client is asked to sign an "Against Medical Advice" form.

  ○ If the client refuses to sign the form, this is also documented by the nurse.

 View Media Supplement: Client Rights (Video)

ADVOCACY

 Overview

- Advocacy refers to nurses' role in supporting clients by ensuring that they are properly informed, that their rights are respected, and that they are receiving the proper level of care.

- Advocacy is one of the most important roles of the nurse, especially when clients are unable to speak or act for themselves.

- Nurses must act as advocates even when they disagree with clients' decisions.

- Today's complex health care system puts clients in a vulnerable position, and nurses are their voice when the system is not acting in their best interest.

- The nursing profession also has a responsibility to support and advocate for legislation that promotes public policies that protect clients as consumers and create a safe environment for their care.

Nursing Role in Advocacy

- As advocates, nurses must ensure that clients are informed of their rights and have adequate information on which to base health care decisions.

- Nurses must be careful to "assist" clients with making health care decisions and not "direct" or "control" their decisions.

- Nurses may need to mediate on the client's behalf when the actions of others are not in the client's best interest or changes need to be made in the plan of care.

- Situations in which nurses may need to advocate for clients or assist them to advocate for themselves include:

  o End-of-life decisions

  o Access to health care

  o Protection of client privacy

  o Informed consent

  o Substandard practice

- Nurses are accountable for their actions even if they are carrying out a provider's prescription. It is the nurse's responsibility to question a provider's prescription if it could harm a client (incorrect dosage for a medication, potential adverse interaction with another prescribed medication, contraindication due to a client allergy or medical history)

ESSENTIAL COMPONENTS OF ADVOCACY	
SKILLS	VALUES
• Risk taking • Vision • Self-confidence • Articulate communication • Assertiveness	• Caring • Autonomy • Respect • Empowerment

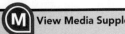 **View Media Supplement:**   Client Advocacy (Video)

INFORMED CONSENT

 Overview

- Informed consent is a legal process by which a client has given written permission for a procedure or treatment to be performed. Consent is considered to be informed when the client has been provided with and understands:

  o   The reason the treatment or procedure is needed

  o   How the treatment or procedure will benefit the client

  o   The risks involved if the client chooses to receive treatment or procedure

  o   Other options to treat the problem, including the option of not treating the problem

- The nurse's role in the informed consent process is to witness the client's signature on the informed consent form and to ensure that informed consent has been appropriately obtained.

Informed Consent Guidelines

- Consent is required for all care given in a health care facility. For most aspects of nursing care, "implied consent" is adequate. The client provides implied consent when the client complies with the instructions provided by the nurse. For example, the nurse is preparing to administer a TB skin test, and the client holds out her arm for the nurse.

- For an invasive procedure or surgery, the client is required to provide written consent.

- State laws prescribe who is able to give informed consent. Laws vary regarding age limitations and emergencies. Nurses are responsible for knowing the laws in the state of practice.

- Signing an Informed Consent Form

  o   The form for informed consent must be signed by a competent adult.

  o   The person who signs the form must be capable of understanding the information provided by the health care professional who will be providing the service and the person must be able to fully communicate in return with the heath care professional.

  o   When the person giving the informed consent is unable to communicate due to a language barrier or hearing impairment, a trained medical interpreter must be provided. Many health care agencies contract with professional interpreters who have additional skills in medical terminology to assist with providing information.

- Individuals authorized to grant consent for another person include:

  o   Parent of a minor

  o   Legal guardian

  o   Court-specified representative

  o   Spouse or closest available relative who has durable power of attorney for health care

- Emancipated minors (minors who are independent from their parents, such as a married minor) can provide informed consent for themselves.

- The nurse must verify that consent is "informed" and witness the client sign the consent form.

RESPONSIBILITIES FOR INFORMED CONSENT		
THE PROVIDER	THE CLIENT	THE NURSE

Obtains informed consent. To do so, the provider must give the client:
• A complete description of the treatment/procedure
• A description of the professionals who will be performing and participating in the treatment
• A description of the potential harm, pain, and/or discomfort that might occur
• Options for other treatments
• The right to refuse treatment
	Gives informed consent. To give informed consent, the client must:
	• Give it voluntarily (no coercion involved).
	• Be competent and of legal age or be an emancipated minor (if the client is unable to provide consent, an authorized person must give consent).
	• Receive enough information to make a decision based on an understanding of what is expected.
		Witnesses informed consent. This means the nurse is responsible for:
		• Ensuring that the provider gave the client the necessary information
		• Ensuring that the client understood the information and is competent to give informed consent
		• Having the client sign the informed consent document
		• Notifying the provider if the client has more questions or appears not to understand any of the information provided (The provider is then responsible for giving clarification.)
		• Documenting:
		  ○ Reinforcement of information originally given by the provider
		  ○ That questions the client had were forwarded to the provider
		  ○ Use of an interpreter

ADVANCE DIRECTIVES

 Overview

- The purpose of advance directives is to communicate a client's wishes regarding end-of-life care should the client become unable to do so.

- The Patient Self-Determination Act (PSDA) requires that all clients admitted to a health care facility be asked if they have advance directives.

    - A client without advance directives must be given written information that outlines her rights related to health care decisions and how to formulate advance directives.

    - A health care representative should be available to help with this process.

- Two components of an advance directive are the living will and the durable power of attorney for health care.

Components of Advance Directives

- Living Will

    ○ A living will is a legal document that expresses the client's wishes regarding medical treatment in the event the client becomes incapacitated and is facing end-of-life issues. Types of treatments that are often addressed in a living will are those that have the capacity to prolong life. Examples of treatments that are addressed are cardiopulmonary resuscitation, mechanical ventilation, and feeding by artificial means.

    ○ Living wills are legal in all states; however, both state statutes and individual health care facility policies may vary. Nurses need to be familiar with their state statute and facility policies.

    ○ Most state laws include provisions that health care providers who follow the health care directive in a living will are protected from liability.

 View Media Supplement: Advance Directive (Image)

- Durable Power of Attorney for Health Care

    ○ A durable power of attorney for health care is a legal document that designates a health care proxy, who is an individual authorized to make health care decisions for a client who is unable. The person who serves in the role of health care proxy to make decisions for the client should be very familiar with the client's wishes. Living wills may be difficult to interpret, especially in the face of unexpected circumstances. A durable power of attorney for health care, as an adjunct to a living, will may be a more effective way of ensuring that the client's decisions about health care are honored.

- Provider's Orders

  o Unless a "do not resuscitate" (DNR) or "allow natural death" (AND) order is written, the nurse should initiate CPR when a client has no pulse or respirations. The written order for a DNR or AND must be placed in the client's medical record. The provider consults the client and the family prior to administering a DNR or AND.

  o Additional orders by the primary care provider are based on the client's individual needs and decisions and provide for comfort measures to relieve symptoms. The client's decision is respected in regard to the use of antibiotics, initiation of diagnostic tests, and provision of nutrition by artificial means.

Nursing Role in Advance Directives

- Nursing responsibilities regarding advance directives include:

  o Providing written information regarding advance directives

  o Documenting the client's advance directives status

  o Ensuring that advance directives are current and reflective of the client's current decisions

  o Informing all members of the health care team of the client's advance directives

CONFIDENTIALITY AND INFORMATION SECURITY

 Overview

- Clients have the right to privacy and confidentiality in relation to their health care information and medical recommendations.

- Nurses who disclose client information to an unauthorized person can be liable for invasion of privacy, defamation, or slander.

- The security and privacy rules of the Health Insurance Portability and Accountability Act (HIPAA) were enacted to protect the confidentiality of health care information and to give the client the right to control the release of information. Specific rights provided by the legislation includes:

  o The rights of clients to obtain a copy of their medical record and to submit requests for changes to the record

  o A requirement for health care providers and insurance providers to provide written information about how medical information is used and how it is shared with other entities (permission must be obtained before information is shared)

Nursing Role in Confidentiality

- It is essential for nurses to be aware of the rights of clients' in regard to privacy and confidentiality. Facility policies and procedures are established in order to ensure compliance with HIPAA regulations. It is essential that nurses know and adhere to the policies and procedures. HIPAA regulations also provide for penalties in the event of noncompliance with the regulations.

- The Privacy Rule of HIPAA requires that nurses protect all written and verbal communication about clients. Components of the privacy rule include:

  o Only health care team members directly responsible for the client's care should be allowed access to the client's records. Nurses may not share information with other clients or staff not involved in the care of the client.

  o Clients have a right to read and obtain a copy of their medical record, and agency policy should be followed when the client requests to read or have a copy of the record.

  o No part of the client chart can be copied except for authorized exchange of documents between health care institutions, for example:

    ▪ Transfer from a hospital to an extended care facility

    ▪ Exchange of documents between a general practitioner and a specialist during a consult

  o Client medical records must be kept in a secure area to prevent inappropriate access to the information. Using public display boards to list client names and diagnoses is restricted.

  o Electronic records should be password protected and care must also be taken to prevent public viewing of the information.

    ▪ Health care workers should use only their own passwords to access information.

  o Client information may not be disclosed to unauthorized individuals/family members who request it or individuals who call on the phone.

    ▪ Many hospitals use a code system in which information is only disclosed to individuals who can provide the code.

    ▪ Nurses should ask any individual inquiring about a client's status for the code and disclose information only when an individual can give the code.

  o Communication about a client should only take place in a private setting where it cannot be overheard by unauthorized individuals. The practice of "walking rounds," where other clients and visitors can hear what is being said, is no longer sanctioned. Taped rounds are also discouraged as nurses should not receive information about clients for whom they are not responsible. Change-of-shift reports can be done at the bedside as long as the client does not have a roommate and no unsolicited visitors are present.

- Information Security

  o Health information systems (HIS) are used to manage administrative functions and clinical functions. The clinical portion of the system is often referred to as the clinical information systems (CIS). The CIS may be used to coordinate essential aspects of client care.

  o In order to comply with HIPAA regulations, each health care facility has specific policies and procedures designed to monitor staff adherence, technical protocols, computer privacy, and data safety.

  o Information security protocols include:

    ▪ Logging off from the computer before leaving the workstation to ensure that others cannot view protected health information (PHI) on the monitor

    ▪ Never sharing a user ID or password with anyone

    ▪ Never leaving a client's chart or other printed or written PHI where others can access it

    ▪ Shredding any printed or written client information used for reporting or client care after it is no longer needed

LEGAL PRACTICE

 Overview

- In order to be safe practitioners, nurses must understand the legal aspects of the nursing profession.

- Understanding the laws governing nursing practice allows nurses to protect client rights and to reduce the risk of nursing liability.

- Nurses are accountable for practicing nursing in accordance with the various sources of law affecting nursing practice. It is important that nurses know and comply with these laws. By practicing nursing within the confines of the law, nurses are able to:

  o Provide safe competent care.

  o Advocate for clients' rights.

  o Provide care that is within the nurse's scope of practice.

  o Discern the responsibilities of nursing in relation to the responsibilities of other members of the health care team.

  o Provide care that is consistent with established standards of care.

  o Shield oneself from liability.

Sources of Law

- Federal Regulations

  - Federal regulations have a great impact on nursing practice. Some of the federal laws impacting nursing practice include:

    - The Health Insurance Portability and Accountability Act (HIPAA)

    - The Americans with Disabilities Act (ADA)

    - The Mental Health Parity Act (MHPA)

    - The Patient Self-Determination Act (PSDA)

    - The Uniform Anatomical Gift Act and the National Organ Transplant Act

- Criminal and Civil Laws

  - Criminal law is a subsection of public law and relates to the relationship of an individual with the government. Violations of criminal law may be categorized as either a felony (a serious crime, such as homicide) or misdemeanor (a less serious crime, such as petty theft). A nurse who falsifies a record to cover up a serious mistake may be found guilty of breaking a criminal law.

  - Civil laws protect the individual rights of people. One type of civil law that relates to the provision of nursing care is tort law. Torts may be classified as unintentional, quasi-intentional, or intentional. Negligence and malpractice (professional negligence) are unintentional torts.

UNINTENTIONAL TORTS	EXAMPLE
Negligence	A nurse fails to implement safety measures for a client who has been identified as at risk for falls.
Malpractice (Professional negligence)	A nurse administers a large dose of medication due to a calculation error. The client has a cardiac arrest and dies.
QUASI-INTENTIONAL TORTS	**EXAMPLE**
Breach of confidentiality	A nurse releases the medical diagnosis of a client to a member of the press.
Defamation of character	A nurse tells a coworker that she believes a client has been unfaithful to the spouse.
INTENTIONAL TORTS	**EXAMPLE**
Assault	The conduct of one person makes another person fearful and apprehensive (threatening to place a nasogastric tube in a client who is refusing to eat).
Battery	Intentional and wrongful physical contact with a person that involves an injury or offensive contact (restraining a client and administering an injection against his wishes).
False imprisonment	A person is confined or restrained against his will (using restraints on a competent client to prevent his leaving the health care facility).

- State Laws

  o The core of nursing practice is regulated by state law.

  o Each state has enacted statutes that define the parameters of nursing practice and give the authority to regulate the practice of nursing to its state board of nursing.

    ■ Boards of nursing have the authority to adopt rules and regulations that further regulate nursing practice. Although the practice of nursing is similar among states, it is critical that nurses know the laws and rules governing nursing in the state in which they practice.

    ■ The laws and rules governing nursing practice in a specific state may be accessed at the state board's Web site.

    ■ Boards of nursing have the authority to both issue and revoke a nursing license.

    ■ Boards also set standards for nursing programs and further delineate the scope of practice for registered nurses, licensed practical nurses, and advanced practice nurses.

  o State laws vary as to when an individual may begin practicing nursing. Some states allow graduates of nursing programs to practice under a limited license, whereas some states require licensure by passing the NCLEX® before working.

- Licensure

  o Until the year 2000, nurses were required to hold a current license in every state in which they practiced. This became problematic with the increase in the electronic practice of nursing. For example, a nurse in one state interprets the reading of a cardiac monitor and provides intervention for a client who is physically located in another state. Additionally, many nurses cross state lines to provide direct care. For example, a nurse who is located near a state border makes home visits on both sides of the state line.

  o To address these issues, the mutual recognition model of nurse licensure (the nurse licensure compact) has been adopted by many states. This model allows nurses who reside in a compact state to practice in another compact state. Nurses must practice in accordance with the statues and rules of the state in which the care is provided. State boards may prohibit a nurse from practicing under the compact if the license of the nurse has been restricted by a board of nursing.

  o Nurses who do not reside in a compact state must practice under the state-based practice model. In other words, if a nurse resides in a non-compact state, the nurse must maintain a current license in every state in which the nurse practices. Currently, some states now require background checks with licensure renewal. It is illegal to practice nursing with an expired license.

Standards of Care (Practice)

- Nurses base practice on established standards of care or legal guidelines for care. These standards of care can be found in:

  o The nurse practice act of each state

    - These acts govern nursing practice, and legal guidelines for practice are established and enforced through a state board of nursing or other government agency.

    - Nurse practice acts vary from state to state, making it obligatory for the nurse to be informed about her state's nurse practice act as it defines the legal parameters of practice.

  o Published standards of nursing practice

    - These are developed by professional organizations and specialty groups, including the American Nurses Association (ANA), the American Association of Critical Care Nurses (AACN), and the American Association of Occupational Health Nurses (AAOHN).

  o Health care facility policies and procedures

    - Policies and procedures, maintained in the facility's policy and procedure manual, establish the standard of practice for employees of that institution.

    - These manuals provide detailed information about how the nurse should respond to or provide care in specific situations and while performing client care procedures.

    - Nurses who practice according to institutional policy are legally protected if that standard of care still results in an injury.

      □ If, for example, a client files a complaint with the board of nursing or seeks legal counsel, the nurse who has followed the facility's policies will not usually be charged with misconduct.

    - It is very important that nurses are familiar with their institution's policies and procedures and provide client care in accordance with these policies. For example:

      □ Assess and document client findings postoperatively according to institutional policy.

      □ Change IV tubing and flush saline locks according to institutional policy.

- Standards of care guide, define, and direct the level of care that should be given by practicing nurses, and they are used in malpractice lawsuits to determine if that level was maintained.

- Nurses should refuse to practice beyond the legal scope of practice and/or outside of their areas of competence regardless of reason (staffing shortage, lack of appropriate personnel).

- Nurses should use the formal chain of command to verbalize concerns related to assignment in light of current legal scope of practice, job description, and area of competence.

Professional Negligence

- Professional negligence is the failure of a person with professional training to act in a reasonable and prudent manner. The terms "reasonable and prudent" are generally used to describe a person who has the average judgment, foresight, intelligence, and skill that would be expected of a person with similar training and experience.

- Negligence issues that prompt most malpractice suits include failure to:

  o Follow either professional or facility established standards of care.

  o Use equipment in a responsible and knowledgeable manner.

  o Communicate effectively and thoroughly with the client.

  o Document care that was provided.

THE FIVE ELEMENTS NECESSARY TO PROVE NEGLIGENCE		
ELEMENT OF LIABILITY	EXPLANATION	EXAMPLE: CLIENT WHO IS A FALL RISK
1. Duty to provide care as defined by a standard	Care that should be given or what a reasonably prudent nurse would do	The nurse should complete a fall risk assessment for all clients upon admission, per facility protocol.
2. Breach of duty by failure to meet standard	Failure to give the standard of care that should have been given	The nurse does not perform a fall risk assessment during admission.
3. Foreseeability of harm	Knowledge that failing to give the proper standard of care may cause harm to the client	The nurse should know that failure to take fall risk precautions may endanger a client at risk for falls.
4. Breach of duty has potential to cause harm (combines elements 2 and 3)	Failure to meet the standard had potential to cause harm – relationship must be provable	If a fall risk assessment is not performed, the client's risk for falls is not determined and the proper precautions are not put in place.
5. Harm occurs	The occurrence of actual harm to the client	The client falls out of bed and breaks his hip.

- Nurses can avoid being liable for negligence by:

  o Following standards of care

  o Giving competent care

  o Communicating with other health team members

  o Developing a caring rapport with clients

  o Fully documenting assessments, interventions, and evaluations

Impaired Coworkers

- Impaired health care providers pose a significant risk to client safety.

- A nurse who suspects a coworker of using alcohol or drugs while working has a duty to report the coworker to appropriate management personnel as specified by institutional policy. At the time of the infraction, the report may need to be made to the immediate supervisor such as the charge nurse to ensure client safety.

- Health care facility policies should provide guidelines for handling employees with a chemical abuse issue, and many provide peer assistance programs that facilitate the health care provider's entry into a treatment program.

- Each state board of nursing has laws and regulations that govern the disposition of nurses who have been reported secondary to chemical abuse. Depending on the individual case, the boards may have the option to require the nurse enter a treatment program, during which time the nurse's license may be retained, suspended, or revoked. If a nurse is allowed to maintain licensure, there are usually work restrictions put in place, such as working in noncritical care areas and being restricted from administering controlled medications.

- Health care providers who are found guilty of misappropriation of controlled substances can also be charged with a criminal offense consistent with the infraction.

- Behaviors consistent with chemical abuse that should be considered suspicious include:

    o Smell of alcohol on breath or frequent use of strong mouthwash or mints

    o Impaired coordination, sleepiness, shakiness, and/or slurred speech

    o Bloodshot eyes

    o Mood swings and memory loss

    o Neglect of personal appearance

    o Excessive use of sick leave, tardiness, or absences after a weekend off, holiday, or payday

    o Frequent requests to leave the unit for short periods of time or to leave the shift early

    o Frequently "forgetting" to have another nurse witness wasting of a controlled substance

    o Frequent involvement in incidences where a client assigned to the nurse reports not receiving pain medication or adequate pain relief (impaired nurse provides questionable explanations)

    o Documenting administration of pain medication to a client who did not receive it or documenting a higher dosage than has been given by other nurses

    o Preferring to work the night shift where supervision is less or on units where controlled substances are more frequently given

- Behaviors may be difficult to detect if the impaired nurse is experienced at masking the addiction.

Mandatory Reporting

- In certain situations, health care providers have a legal obligation to report their findings in accordance with state law.

- Abuse

  o All 51 jurisdictions (the 50 states and the District of Colombia) have statutes requiring report of suspicion of child abuse. The statutes set out which occupations are mandatory reporters. In many states, nurses are mandatory reporters.

  o A number of states also mandate that health care providers, including nurses, report suspected abuse of the older adults and dependent adults.

  o Nurses are mandated to report any suspicion of abuse following facility policy.

- Communicable Diseases

  o Nurses are also mandated to report to the proper agency (local health department, state health department) when a client has been diagnosed with a communicable disease.

  o A complete list of reportable diseases and a description of the reporting system are available through the Centers for Disease Control and Prevention Web site, www.cdc.gov. Each state mandates which diseases must be reported in that state. There are more than 60 communicable diseases that must be reported to public health departments to allow officials to:

    ▪ Ensure appropriate medical treatment of diseases (tuberculosis).

    ▪ Monitor for common-source outbreaks (foodborne – hepatitis A).

    ▪ Plan and evaluate control and prevention plans (immunizations for preventable diseases).

    ▪ Identify outbreaks and epidemics.

    ▪ Determine public health priorities based on trends.

    ▪ Educate the community on prevention and treatment of these diseases.

Organ Donation

- Organ and tissue donation is regulated by federal and state laws. Health care facilities have policies and procedures to guide health care workers involved with organ donation.

- Donations may be stipulated in a will or designated on an official card.

- Federal law requires health care facilities to provide access to trained specialists who make the request to clients and/or family members and provide information regarding consent, organ and tissues that can be donated, and how burial or cremation will be impacted by donation.

- Nurses are responsible for answering questions regarding the donation process and for providing emotional support to family members.

Transcribing Medical Prescriptions

- Nurses may need to receive new prescriptions for client care or medications after a provider has left the institution or the client has exhibited a change in status.

- When transcribing a prescription into a paper or electronic chart, nurses must:

  - Be sure to include all necessary elements of a prescription (date and time prescription was written, new client care prescription or medication including dosage, frequency, route of administration, and signature of nurse transcribing the prescription as well as the provider who verbally gave the prescription).

  - Follow institutional policy with regard to the time frame within which the provider must sign the order (usually within 24 hours).

  - Use strategies to prevent errors when taking a medical prescription that is given verbally or over the phone by the primary care provider.

    - Repeat back the prescription given, making sure to include the medication name (spell if necessary), dosage, time, and route.

    - Question any prescription that may seem contraindicated due to a previous or concurrent prescription or client condition.

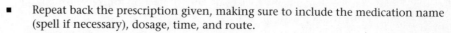

ETHICAL PRACTICE

 Overview

- Ethics has several definitions, but the foundation of ethics is based on an expected behavior of a certain group in relation to what is considered right and wrong.

- Morals are the values and beliefs held by a person that guides behavior and decision making.

- Ethical theory analyzes varying philosophies, systems, ideas, and principles used to make judgments about what is right and wrong and good and bad. Two common types of ethical theory are utilitarianism and deontology.

- Ethical principles are standards of what is right or wrong with regard to important social values and norms. Ethical principles pertaining to the treatment of clients include:

  - Autonomy – the ability of the client to make personal decisions, even when those decisions may not be in the client's own best interest

  - Beneficence – the care that is in the best interest of the client

  - Fidelity – keeping one's promise to the client about care that was offered

  - Justice – fair treatment in matters related to physical and psychosocial care and use of resources

  - Nonmaleficence – prevention of harm or pain as much as possible during treatment

- Unusual or complex ethical issues may need to be dealt with by a hospital's ethics committee.

Ethical Decision Making in Nursing

- Ethical dilemmas are problems for which more than one choice can be made and the choice is influenced by the values and beliefs of the decision makers. These are common in health care, and nurses must be prepared to apply ethical theory and decision making.

- A problem is an ethical dilemma if:

  - It cannot be solved solely by a review of scientific data.

  - It involves a conflict between two moral imperatives.

  - The answer will have profound effect on the situation/client.

- Nurses have a responsibility to be advocates and identify and report ethical situations.

  - Doing so through the chain of command offers some protection against retribution.

  - Some state nurse associations offer protection for nurses who report substandard or unethical practice.

- Ethical decision making is the process by which a decision is made about an ethical issue. Frequently, this requires that a balance be struck between science and morality. There are several steps in ethical decision making:

  - Identify whether the issue is indeed an ethical dilemma.

  - State the ethical dilemma including all surrounding issues and individuals involved.

  - List and analyze all possible options for resolving the dilemma and review implications of each option.

  - Select the option that is in concert with the ethical principle applicable to this situation, the decision maker's values and beliefs, and the profession's values set forth for client care. Justify why that one option was selected.

  - Apply this decision to the dilemma and evaluate the outcomes.

- The *American Nurses Association Code of Ethics for Nurses* (2001) and the *International Council of Nurses' Code of Ethics for Nurses* (2006) are documents commonly used by professional nurses. The Code of Ethics for Licensed Practical/Vocational Nurses issued by the National Association for Practical Nurse Education and Services also serves as a set of standards for Nursing Practice. Codes of ethics are available at the organizations' Web sites.

- The Uniform Determination of Death Act (UDDA) is a document that can be used to assist with end-of-life and organ donor issues.

  - The UDDA provides two formal definitions of death that were developed by the National Conference of Commissioners on Uniform State Laws. Death is determined by one of two criteria:

    - An irreversible cessation of circulatory and respiratory functions

    - Irreversible cessation of all functions of the entire brain, including the brain stem

  - A determination of death must be made in accordance with accepted medical standards.

THE NURSE'S ROLE IN ETHICAL DECISION MAKING	
NURSE'S ROLE	**EXAMPLES**
An agent for the client facing an ethical decision	• Caring for an adolescent client who has to decide whether or not to undergo an abortion even though her parents believe it is wrong • Discussing options with a parent who has to decide whether or not to consent to a blood transfusion for a child when their religion prohibits such treatment
A decision maker in regard to nursing practice	• Assigning staff nurses a higher client load than recommended because administration has cut the number of nurses per shift • Witnessing a surgeon discuss only surgical options with a client without informing the client about more conservative measures available

CHAPTER 3: PROFESSIONAL RESPONSIBILITIES

(A) Application Exercises

1. Which of the following is an infraction of the Privacy Rules outlined by HIPAA? (Select all that apply.)

_____ Reviewing the chart of a client assigned to another nurse

_____ Making a copy of a client's most current laboratory results for the primary care provider during rounds

_____ Answering questions about a client's condition for the client's daughter

_____ Discussing a client's condition over the phone with an individual who has provided the client's information code

_____ Participating in walking rounds that involve the exchange of information outside clients' rooms

2. A client who is scheduled for surgery is brought to the surgical unit. The client hands the nurse the information about advance directives he received from the admitting nurse and says, "Here, I don't know why she gave me this stuff. I'm too young to worry about what life-sustaining measures I want done for me." Which of the following actions should the nurse take next?

A. Take the papers and send them back to the admitting department with a note stating that the client does not wish to address this issue at this time.

B. Explain to the client that you never know what can happen during surgery and that he should fill the papers out "just in case."

C. Contact a client representative to talk with the client and offer additional information about the purpose of advance directives.

D. Inform the client that surgery cannot be conducted unless he completes the advance directives forms.

3. In which of the following situations should a nurse act as a client advocate? (Select all that apply.)

_____ Verifying that a client understands what is done during a cardiac catheterization

_____ Discussing treatment options for a terminal diagnosis

_____ Informing members of the health care team that a client has DNR status

_____ Reporting that a health team member on the previous shift did not provide care as prescribed

_____ Assisting a client to make a decision about his care based on the nurse's recommendations

4. Which of the following outlines the rights of individuals in health care settings?

A. ANA Code of Ethics

B. HIPAA

C. Patient Self-Determination Act

D. Patient Care Partnership

5. A nurse reviewing a client's chart discovers that the client's DNR order has expired. The client's condition has not been stable today. Which of the following actions should the nurse take?

    A. Assume that the client still wishes to be a DNR client and anticipate no action if she goes into cardiopulmonary arrest.

    B. Write a note on the front of the provider order sheet asking that the DNR order be reordered.

    C. Anticipate that CPR will be instituted if the client goes into cardiopulmonary arrest.

    D. Call the primary care provider to get the order immediately reinstated.

6. An 18-year-old client in the emergency department has been diagnosed with acute appendicitis with a recommendation for an immediate appendectomy. The client begins to put his clothes on, saying he does not want to have surgery and is going home. Which of the following actions should the nurse take prior to the client leaving the facility?

    A. Validate that the client understands the consequences, including the possibility of death.

    B. Complete an incident form outlining the facts surrounding the occurrence.

    C. Ask security to detain the client until a legally responsible person can sign the surgical permit.

    D. Do nothing and let the client leave without incident due to his right to refuse treatment.

7. A toddler is being treated in the emergency department following a head contusion from a fall. History reveals the toddler lives at home with only her mother. The provider's discharge instructions include waking the child up every hour during the night to assess for signs of a possible head injury. In which of the following situations should the nurse intervene and attempt to prevent discharge?

    A. The mother states she does not have insurance or money for a follow-up visit.

    B. The child states her head hurts and she wants to go home.

    C. The nurse smells alcohol on the mother's breath.

    D. The mother verbalizes fear about taking the child home and requests she be kept overnight.

8. A newly licensed nurse is preparing to insert an intravenous catheter in a client. While she has done this twice in nursing school, she would feel more confident if she could review the procedure again before insertion. Which of the following sources should the nurse use to obtain this information and the standard at which it should be performed?

    A. Internet site

    B. Institutional policy and procedure manual

    C. Charge nurse

    D. Nurse practice act

9. A nurse witnesses an assistive personnel (AP) under her supervision reprimanding a client for not using the urinal properly. The AP threatens to put a diaper on the client if he does not use the urinal more carefully next time. Which of the following torts is the AP committing?

    A. Assault

    B. Battery

    C. False imprisonment

    D. Invasion of privacy

CHAPTER 3: PROFESSIONAL RESPONSIBILITIES

 Application Exercises Answer Key

1. Which of the following is an infraction of the Privacy Rules outlined by HIPAA? (Select all that apply.)

   __X__   **Reviewing the chart of a client assigned to another nurse**

   __X__   **Making a copy of a client's most current laboratory results for the primary care provider during rounds**

   __X__   **Answering questions about a client's condition for the client's daughter**

   _____   Discussing a client's condition over the phone with an individual who has provided the client's information code

   __X__   **Participating in walking rounds that involve the exchange of information outside clients' rooms**

    Discussing a client's condition over the phone with an individual who has provided the client's information code is allowed by HIPAA. Many health care institutions use a code system to determine who should have access to a client's health care information. All of the other options could allow inappropriate dissemination of client information.

 NCLEX® Connection: Management of Care, Confidentiality/Information Security

2. A client who is scheduled for surgery is brought to the surgical unit. The client hands the nurse the information about advance directives he received from the admitting nurse and says, "Here, I don't know why she gave me this stuff. I'm too young to worry about what life-sustaining measures I want done for me." Which of the following actions should the nurse take next?

   A. Take the papers and send them back to the admitting department with a note stating that the client does not wish to address this issue at this time.

   B. Explain to the client that you never know what can happen during surgery and that he should fill the papers out "just in case."

   C. Contact a client representative to talk with the client and offer additional information about the purpose of advance directives.

   D. Inform the client that surgery cannot be conducted unless he completes the advance directives forms.

   It is important that the client be properly informed about the purpose of advance directives and their role in protecting his rights. While the client is not required to fill out the papers, his comments indicate he might not understand their purpose, and the nurse must advocate for him to ensure his rights are protected. The nurse, however, should never coerce a client into signing any legal forms, even if she believes it would be in the client's best interest.

 NCLEX® Connection: Management of Care, Advance Directives

3. In which of the following situations should a nurse act as a client advocate? (Select all that apply.)

   __X__   **Verifying that a client understands what is done during a cardiac catheterization**

   _____   Discussing treatment options for a terminal diagnosis

   __X__   **Informing members of the health care team that a client has DNR status**

   __X__   **Reporting that a health team member on the previous shift did not provide care as prescribed**

   _____   Assisting a client to make a decision about his care based on the nurse's recommendations

As an advocate, a nurse must ensure that clients are informed of their rights and have adequate information upon which to base health care decisions. Verifying that a client understands what will be done during an invasive procedure ensures that a client has made an informed decision to consent to the procedure. It is also the nurse's responsibility to ensure that staff are providing proper care and are aware that a DNR client may be a part of that care. Discussing treatment options and making recommendations for care are not within the nurse's scope of practice.

 NCLEX® Connection: Management of Care, Advocacy

4. Which of the following outlines the rights of individuals in health care settings?

   A. ANA Code of Ethics

   B. HIPAA

   C. Patient Self-Determination Act

   D. Patient Care Partnership

The rights of individuals in health care settings is outlined in the Patient Care Partnership, which is a document written in plain language and translated to several languages for non-English speakers. The ANA Code of Ethics provides professional standards that have been developed by the American Nurses Association for nurses in an effort to provide a set of principles to aid in ethical problem solving. HIPAA, or the Privacy Rule of the Health Insurance Portability and Accountability Act, is a law that requires nurses to protect all written and verbal communication about clients. The Patient Self-Determination Act is federal legislation that requires all clients admitted to a health care facility to be asked if they have advance directives.

 NCLEX® Connection: Management of Care, Client Rights

5. A nurse reviewing a client's chart discovers that the client's DNR order has expired. The client's condition has not been stable today. Which of the following actions should the nurse take?

    A. Assume that the client still wishes to be a DNR client and anticipate no action if she goes into cardiopulmonary arrest.

    B. Write a note on the front of the provider order sheet asking that the DNR order be reordered.

    C. Anticipate that CPR will be instituted if the client goes into cardiopulmonary arrest.

    D. Call the primary care provider to get the order immediately reinstated.

DNR prescriptions must be reinstated by the primary care provider on an institutionally specified basis. Without a current DNR prescription, the nurse must institute CPR if the client goes into cardiopulmonary arrest. Since the client has been unstable today, the nurse should call the primary care provider to get a current order reinstituted.

 NCLEX® Connection: Management of Care, Advocacy

6. An 18-year-old client in the emergency department has been diagnosed with acute appendicitis with a recommendation for an immediate appendectomy. The client begins to put his clothes on, saying he does not want to have surgery and is going home. Which of the following actions should the nurse take prior to the client leaving the facility?

    A. Validate that the client understands the consequences, including the possibility of death.

    B. Complete an incident form outlining the facts surrounding the occurrence.

    C. Ask security to detain the client until a legally responsible person can sign the surgical permit.

    D. Do nothing and let the client leave without incident due to his right to refuse treatment.

Clients of legal age for consent (18 years of age) can refuse care at any time for any reason as long as they are not impaired (alcohol, drugs), are competent (of normal intelligence, alert, and oriented), and understand the consequences of the decision. Subsequently, the most important action by the nurse is to make sure the client understands the consequences of his actions. While clients who leave against medical advice are encouraged to sign the relevant form, it is not legally necessary. The nurse, however, should carefully and thoroughly document what information was provided to the client and his response. Asking security to detain the client could be considered false imprisonment. Letting him leave does not ensure that he is making an informed decision.

 NCLEX® Connection: Management of Care, Legal Rights and Responsibilities

7. A toddler is being treated in the emergency department following a head contusion from a fall. History reveals the toddler lives at home with only her mother. The provider's discharge instructions include waking the child up every hour during the night to assess for signs of a possible head injury. In which of the following situations should the nurse intervene and attempt to prevent discharge?

    A. The mother states she does not have insurance or money for a follow-up visit.

    B. The child states her head hurts and she wants to go home.

    C. The nurse smells alcohol on the mother's breath.

    D. The mother verbalizes fear about taking the child home and requests she be kept overnight.

It would be unsafe to send a child who requires hourly monitoring home with a mother who might be chemically impaired. It is the nurse's responsibility to detect possible harm and research other options, such as admission to the facility or the enlistment and aid of another family member. Lack of insurance should not contraindicate discharge, but information should be made available about agencies that can provide follow-up care based on financial need. Education regarding the hourly assessments and provision of the facility's phone number should be provided to help reduce the mother's fear about taking the child home.

 NCLEX® Connection: Management of Care, Legal Rights and Responsibilities

8. A newly licensed nurse is preparing to insert an intravenous catheter in a client. While she has done this twice in nursing school, she would feel more confident if she could review the procedure again before insertion. Which of the following sources should the nurse use to obtain this information and the standard at which it should be performed?

    A. Internet site

    B. Institutional policy and procedure manual

    C. Charge nurse

    D. Nurse practice act

The institutional policy and procedure manual will provide a description of how the procedure should be performed, as well as guidelines regarding the standard of practice set forth by the health care institution. An Internet site may not provide direction consistent with the institution's policy, and the nurse should review the policy directly instead of obtaining the information anecdotally from another nurse. The state's nurse practice act defines the parameters for the legal practice of nursing, but it will not describe how to perform the skill nor the standard at which it is to be performed according to institutional policy.

 NCLEX® Connection: Safety and Infection Control, Error Prevention

9. A nurse witnesses an assistive personnel (AP) under her supervision reprimanding a client for not using the urinal properly. The AP threatens to put a diaper on the client if he does not use the urinal more carefully next time. Which of the following torts is the AP committing?

   A. Assault

   B. Battery

   C. False imprisonment

   D. Invasion of privacy

   By threatening the client, the AP is committing assault. The threats could make the client become fearful and apprehensive. Since the AP has only verbally threatened the client, battery has not occurred. False imprisonment and invasion of privacy have not been committed.

 NCLEX® Connection: Management of Care, Legal Rights and Responsibilities

CHAPTER 4: MAINTAINING A SAFE ENVIRONMENT

- Handling Infectious and Hazardous Materials
- Safe Use of Equipment
- Accident and Injury Prevention
- Home Safety
- Ergonomic Principles

NCLEX® CONNECTIONS

When reviewing the content in this chapter, keep in mind the relevant sections of the NCLEX® outline, in particular:

CLIENT NEEDS: SAFETY AND INFECTION CONTROL

Relevant topics/tasks include:
- Accident/Injury Prevention
  - ○ Make an appropriate room assignment for the cognitively impaired client.
- Error Prevention
  - ○ Verify appropriateness and/or accuracy of a treatment order.
- Handling Hazardous and Infectious Materials
  - ○ Follow procedures for handling biohazardous materials.
- Home Safety
  - ○ Evaluate client care environment for fire/environmental hazards.
- Safe Use of Equipment
  - ○ Facilitate appropriate and safe use of equipment.

Chapter 4	Maintaining a Safe Environment

 Overview

- Maintaining a safe environment refers to the precautions and considerations required to ensure that physical environments are safe for both clients and staff.

- Knowing how to maintain client safety has been identified by the Institute of Medicine as a competency that graduates of nursing programs must possess.

- Quality and Safety Education for Nurses (QSEN) faculty propose that nursing education focus not only on the knowledge needed to provide safe care but also on the skills and attitudes that accompany this competency.

- To maintain a safe environment, nurses must have knowledge, skills, and attitude about:

  o   Handling Infectious and Hazardous Materials

  o   Safe Use of Equipment

  o   Accident and Injury Prevention

  o   Home Safety

  o   Ergonomic Principles

HANDLING INFECTIOUS AND HAZARDOUS MATERIALS

 Overview

- Handling infectious and hazardous materials refers both to infection control procedures and to precautions for handling toxic, radioactive, or other hazardous materials.

- These safety measures are taken to protect the client, nurse, and other personnel and individuals from harmful materials and organisms.

- There are four levels of precautions (standard, airborne, droplet, contact) recommended for individuals coming in contact with clients carrying infectious organisms. Precautions consistent with the infectious organism should be followed as indicated.

- A manual containing material safety data sheets (MSDS) should be available in every workplace and should provide safety information such as level of toxicity, handling and storage guidelines, and first aid and containment measures to take in case of accidental release of toxic, radioactive, or other dangerous materials. This manual should be available to all employees and may be housed in a location such as the emergency department of a hospital.

Infection Control

- Infection control is extremely important to prevent cross contamination of communicable organisms and health care-associated infections.

  o Staff education on infection prevention and control is a responsibility of the nurse.

  o Facility policies and procedures should serve as a resource for proper implementation of infection prevention and control.

  o Clients suspected of, or diagnosed with, a communicable disease should be placed in the appropriate form of isolation.

  o The nurse should ensure that appropriate equipment is available and that isolation procedures are properly carried out by all health care team members.

  o Use of standard precautions by all members of the health care team should be enforced. Employees who are allergic to latex should have nonlatex gloves made available to them.

  o Hand hygiene facilities, as well as hand sanitizer, must be readily accessible to employees in client care areas.

  o Sturdy, moisture-resistant bags (usually red in color) should be used for soiled items, and the bags should be tied securely with a knot at the top. Double bagging is not cost effective and is unnecessary unless the outside of a bag becomes contaminated.

  o Retractable needles or needles with capping mechanisms, needleless syringes, and IV piggyback tubing with needleless connections should be available for use to prevent accidental needlesticks. Education on how to safely use these devices will prevent misuse during client care and staff injuries from improper manipulation.

  o Sharps containers should be readily available in client care areas, and any needlestick involving an employee should be reported in accordance with facility policy and state law. An incident or occurrence report should also be filed. Most policies include testing of the client and nurse for bloodborne illnesses such as hepatitis and human immunodeficiency virus (HIV).

Hazardous Materials

- Nurses and other members of the health care team are at risk for exposure to hazardous materials.

- Employees have the right to refuse to work in hazardous working conditions if there is a clear threat to their health.

- Health care team members should follow occupational safety and health guidelines as set by the Occupational Safety and Health Administration (OSHA). Guidelines include:

  o Providing each employee a work environment that is free from recognized hazards that can cause or are likely to cause death or serious physical harm

  o Making protective gear accessible to employees working under hazardous conditions or with hazardous materials (antineoplastic medications, sterilization chemicals)

○ Providing measurement devices and keeping records that document an employee's level of exposure over time to hazardous materials, such as radiation from x-rays

○ Providing education and recertification opportunities to each employee regarding these rules and regulations, such as handling of hazardous materials

○ Maintaining a manual available to all employees, usually in a central location, that outlines proper procedures for containment of hazardous materials

○ Designating an institutional hazardous materials (HAZMAT) response team that responds to handle and control leaks or spills

Nursing Role in Handling Infectious and Hazardous Materials

- Clean and maintain equipment that is shared by several clients on a unit (blood pressure cuffs, thermometers, pulse oximeters).

- Keep designated equipment in the rooms of clients who are infected with a resistant organism (vancomycin-resistant enterococcus, methicillin-resistant staphylococcus aureus).

- Use standard precautions at all times.

- Employ proper handwashing techniques.

- Use needlestick precautions when administering parenteral medications.

- Maintain knowledge of rules and regulations and proper procedures for handling infectious/hazardous materials (use of red biohazard bag for disposal of contaminated materials, proper use of puncture-proof containers for needles).

SAFE USE OF EQUIPMENT

 Overview

- Safe use of equipment refers to appropriate operation of health care-related equipment by trained staff. Equipment-related injuries may occur as a result of malfunction, disrepair, or mishandling of mechanical equipment.

- Nurses must ensure that they have the competence necessary to use equipment for tasks that fall within their scope of practice. Nurses should only use equipment after receiving sufficient instruction.

- Equipment should be regularly inspected by the engineering or maintenance department and by the user prior to use. Faulty equipment (frayed cords, disrepair) can start a fire or cause an electrical shock and should be removed from use and reported immediately per the health care agency's policy.

Nursing Role in Safe Use of Equipment

- Nurses' responsibilities related to equipment safety include:

○ Learning how to use and maintaining competency in the use of equipment

- ○ Checking that equipment is accurately set and functioning properly (oxygen, nasogastric suction) at the beginning and during each shift

- ○ Ensuring that electrical equipment is grounded (three-pronged plug and grounded outlet) to decrease the risk for electrical shock

- ○ Ensuring that outlet covers are used in environments with individuals at risk for sticking items into them

- ○ Unplugging equipment using the plug, not the cord, to prevent bending the plug prongs, which increases the risk for electrical shock

- ○ Ensuring that life-support equipment is plugged into outlets designated to be powered by a backup generator during power outages

- ○ Disconnecting all electrical equipment prior to cleaning

- ○ Ensuring that all pumps (general and PCA) have free-flow protection to prevent an overdose of fluids or medications (JCAHO, 2004)

- ○ Ensuring that outlets are not overcrowded and extension cords are used only when absolutely necessary (if they must be used in an open area, tape the cords to the floor)

- ○ Using all equipment only as it is intended

- ○ Immediately removing nonworking equipment from the client care area and sending it to the proper department for repair or disposal

ACCIDENT AND INJURY PREVENTION

 Overview

- Preventing injury is a major nursing responsibility. Many factors affect a client's ability to protect himself. Those factors include the client's:

  - ○ Age (the young and the old are at greater risk)

  - ○ Mobility

  - ○ Cognitive and sensory awareness

  - ○ Emotional state

  - ○ Lifestyle and safety awareness

- All health care workers must be aware of:

  - ○ How to assess for and recognize clients at risk for safety issues

  - ○ Procedural safety guidelines

  - ○ Protocols for responding to dangerous situations

  - ○ Security plans

  - ○ Identification and documentation of incidents and responses per health care agency policy

Falls

- Prevention of client falls is a major nursing priority. All clients admitted to health care institutions should be assessed for risk factors related to falls and, based on the assessment, preventative measures should be implemented.

- Older adult clients may be at an increased risk for falls due to decreased strength, impaired mobility and balance, and endurance limitations combined with decreased sensory perception.

- Other clients at increased risk include those with decreased visual acuity, generalized weakness, urinary frequency, gait and balance problems (cerebral palsy, injury, multiple sclerosis) and cognitive dysfunction. Side effects of medications (orthostatic hypotension, drowsiness) can also increase the risk for falls.

- Clients are at greater risk for falls when more than one of the risk factors are present.

- Prevention of Falls

  o Complete a fall risk assessment on the client upon admission and at regular intervals for individualization of the care plan to limit the risk of falls.

  o Document all identified risks and implement specific measures to reduce the risk for falls. The plan for each client is individualized based on the fall risk assessment. For example, if the client has orthostatic hypotension, instruct the client to avoid getting up too quickly, to sit on the side of the bed for a few seconds prior to standing, and to stand at the side of the bed for a few seconds prior to walking. General measures to prevent falls include the following:

    ■ Be sure the client knows how to use the call light, that it is in reach, and encourage its use.

    ■ Respond to call lights in a timely manner.

    ■ Orient the client to the setting (grab bars, call light) and ensure that the client understands how to use all assistive devices and can locate necessary items.

    ■ Place clients at risk for falls near the nursing station.

    ■ Ensure that bedside tables and overbed tables and frequently used items (telephone, water, tissues, call light) are within the client's reach.

    ■ Maintain the bed in low position.

    ■ Keep bed rails up and the bed in the low position for clients who are sedated, unconscious, or otherwise compromised.

    ■ Avoid using full side bed rails for clients who get out of bed or attempt to get out of bed without assistance.

    ■ Provide the client with nonskid footwear.

    ■ Keep the floor free from clutter with a clear path to the bathroom (no scatter rugs, cords, furniture).

    ■ Keep assistive devices (glasses, walkers, transfer devices) nearby after validation of safe use by the client and family.

- Educate the client and family/caregivers on identified risks and the plan of care.

- Lock wheels on beds, wheelchairs, and carts to prevent the device from rolling during transfers or stops.

- Use chair or bed sensors to alert staff of independent ambulation for clients at risk for getting up unattended.

- Report and document all incidents per the health care agency's policy. This provides valuable information that may be helpful in preventing similar incidents.

Seizures

- A seizure is a sudden surge of electrical activity in the brain. Seizures may occur at any time during a person's life and may be due to epilepsy, fever, or a variety of medical conditions. Partial seizures are due to electrical surges in one part of the brain, and generalized seizures involve the entire brain.

- Seizure precautions (measures to protect the client from injury should a seizure occur) are taken for clients who have a history of seizures that involve the entire body and/or result in unconsciousness.

  - Ensure rescue equipment is at the bedside, including oxygen, an oral airway, and suction equipment. A saline lock may be placed for intravenous access if the client is at high risk for experiencing a generalized seizure.

  - Inspect the client's environment for items that may cause injury in the event of a seizure and remove items that are not necessary for current treatment.

  - Assist the client at risk for a seizure with ambulation and transfers to reduce the risk of injury.

  - Advise all caregivers and family not to put anything in the client's mouth in the event of a seizure (except in status epilepticus, where an airway is needed).

  - Advise all caregivers and family not to restrain the client in the event of a seizure. Instead, ensure the client's safety by lowering him to the floor or bed, protecting his head, removing nearby furniture, providing privacy, putting the client on his side with his head slightly flexed forward if possible, and loosening clothing to prevent injury and promote dignity.

  - In the event of a seizure, stay with the client, protect the client from injury, and call for help.

  - Administer medications as prescribed.

  - Note the duration of the seizure and the sequence and type of movement.

  - After a seizure, explain what happened to the client and provide comfort, understanding, and a quiet environment for recovery.

  - Document the seizure in the client's record along with any precipitating behaviors and a description of the event (movements, any injuries, length of seizure, aura, postictal state) and report it to the primary care provider.

Seclusion and Restraints

- Seclusion and restraints are used to prevent clients from injuring themselves or others.

    o Seclusion is the placement of a client in a room that is private, isolated, and safe. This is usually done for clients who are at risk for injuring themselves or others.

    o Physical restraint involves the application of a device that limits the client's movement. A restraint may limit the movement of the entire body or a body part.

    o Chemical restraints are medications used to control the client's disruptive behavior.

- Nurses must recognize that clients can be injured with the use of restraints.

    o Deaths by asphyxiation and strangulation have occurred with restraints.

    o The client may also experience complications related to immobility, such as pressure ulcers, urinary and fecal incontinence, and pneumonia.

- Legal Considerations

    o Nurses should understand agency polices as well as federal and state laws that govern the use of restraints and seclusion.

    o False imprisonment means the confinement of person without his consent. Improper use of restraints may subject the nurse to charges of false imprisonment.

- Guidelines for Seclusion and Restraints

    o In general, seclusion and/or restraints should be ordered for the shortest duration necessary and only if less restrictive measures have proved insufficient. They are for the physical protection of the client or the protection of other clients or staff.

    o A client may voluntarily request temporary seclusion in cases where the environment is disturbing or seems too stimulating.

    o The use of restraints is a difficult adjustment for both the client and the family. The client loses his freedom and may be embarrassed and experience low self-esteem and depression. The nurse can allay some of the concerns by explaining the purpose of the restraint and that the restraint is only temporary.

    o Seclusion and/or restraints must never be used for:

        ▪ Convenience of the staff

        ▪ Punishment for the client

        ▪ Clients who are extremely physically or mentally unstable

        ▪ Clients who cannot tolerate the decreased stimulation of a seclusion room

    o Restraints should:

        ▪ Never interfere with treatment.

        ▪ Restrict movement as little as is necessary to ensure safety.

        ▪ Fit properly.

        ▪ Be easily changed to decrease the chance of injury and to provide for the greatest level of dignity.

NURSING LEADERSHIP AND MANAGEMENT

- When all other less restrictive means have been tried to prevent a client from harming self or others, the following must occur for seclusion or restraints to be used:
  - The treatment must be prescribed by the provider based on a face-to-face assessment of the client.
    - In an emergency situation in which there is immediate risk to the client or others, the nurse may place a client in restraints. The nurse must obtain a prescription from the primary care provided as soon as possible in accordance with agency policy (usually within 1 hr).
  - The prescription must specify the reason for the restraint, the type of restraint, the location of the restraint, how long the restraint may be used, and the type of behaviors demonstrated by the client that warrant use of the restraint.
  - The provider must rewrite the prescription, specifying the type of restraint, every 24 hr or the frequency of time specified by facility policy.
    - PRN prescriptions for restraints are not allowed.
- Nursing responsibilities must be identified in the prescription, including how often the client should be:
  - Assessed (including neurosensory checks, usually at least every 2 hr, of affected extremities: circulation, sensation, mobility)
  - Offered food and fluid
  - Provided with means for hygiene and elimination
  - Monitored for vital signs
  - Offered range of motion of extremities
- The frequency of client assessments with regard to food, fluids, comfort, and safety should be performed and documented every 15 to 30 min.
- Other Nursing Responsibilities
  - Be aware and follow agency polices regarding restraints including the need for a signed consent from the client or guardian.
  - Review the manufacturer's instructions for correct application.
  - Remove or replace restraints frequently to ensure good circulation to the area and allow for full range of motion to the limb that has been restricted.
  - Pad bony prominences.
  - Use a quick release knot to tie the restraint to the bed frame (loose knots that are easily removed) where it will not tighten when the bed is raised or lowered.
  - Ensure that the restraint is loose enough for range of motion and has enough room to fit two fingers between the device and the client to prevent injury.
  - Regularly assess the need for continued use of the restraints to allow for discontinuation at the earliest possible time while ensuring the client's safety.

- Never leave the client unattended without the restraint.
- Document the use of restraints. This must include:
  - The behavior or precipitating events that make the restraint necessary
  - Attempts to use alternatives to restraints and the client's response
  - The client's level of consciousness
  - Type of restraint used and location
  - Education/explanations to the client and family
  - Exact time of application and removal
  - The client's behavior while restrained
  - Type and frequency of care (range of motion, neurosensory checks, removal, integumentary checks)
  - The client's response when the restraint is removed
  - Medication administration

Fire Safety

- Fires in health care facilities are usually due to problems related to electrical or anesthetic equipment. Unauthorized smoking may also be the case of a fire.

- All staff must be instructed in fire response procedures, which include knowing the:

  - Location of exits, fire extinguishers, and oxygen turn-offs valves
  - Evacuation plan for the unit and facility

- Fire response in health care settings always follows the RACE sequence:

  - **Rescue** – Protect and evacuate clients in close proximity to the fire.
  - **Alarm** – Report the fire by sounding the alarm.
  - **Contain** – Contain the fire by closing doors and windows as well as turning off any sources of oxygen. Clients who are on life support are ventilated with a bag-valve mask.
  - **Extinguish** – Extinguish the fire if possible using an appropriate fire extinguisher.
    - There are three classes of fire extinguisher.
      - Class A is for paper, wood, upholstery, rags, or other types of trash fires.
      - Class B is for flammable liquids and gas fires.
      - Class C is for electrical fires.

NURSING LEADERSHIP AND MANAGEMENT

- To use a fire extinguisher, follow the PASS sequence:
    - **P**ull – Pull the pin.
    - **A**im – Aim at the base of the fire.
    - **S**queeze – Squeeze the levers.
    - **S**weep – Sweep the extinguisher from side to side, covering the area of the fire.

HOME SAFETY

 Overview

- In addition to taking measures to prevent injury of clients in a health care setting, nurses play a pivotal role in promoting safety in the client's home and community. Nurses often collaborate with the client, family, and members of the interdisciplinary team (social workers, occupational therapists, physical therapists) to promote the client's safety.

- A number of factors contribute to the client's risk for injury. These factors include the client's:
    - Age and developmental status
    - Mobility and balance
    - Knowledge about safety hazards
    - Sensory and cognitive awareness
    - Communication skills
    - Home and work environment
    - Community

- To initiate a plan of care, the nurse must identify risk factors using a risk assessment tool and complete a nursing history, physical examination, and home hazard appraisal.

Safety Risks Based on Age and Developmental Status

- The age and developmental status of the client creates specific safety risks.

RISK	PREVENTION EDUCATION
	Infants and toddlers
Aspiration	• Keep all small objects out of reach. • Check toys for loose parts. • Do not feed the infant hard candy, peanuts, popcorn, or whole or sliced pieces of hot dog. • Do not place the infant in the supine position while feeding or prop the infant's bottle. • A pacifier (if used) should be constructed of one piece. • Provide parents with information about prevention of lead poisoning.
Suffocation	• Keep plastic bags out of reach. • Make sure crib mattress fits snugly and that crib slats are no more than 23/8 inches apart. • Never leave an infant or toddler alone in the bath tub. • Remove crib toys such as mobiles from over the bed as soon as infant begins to push up. • Keep latex balloons away from infants and toddlers. • Fence swimming pools and use a locked gate. • Begin swimming lessons when the child's developmental status allows for protective responses such as closing mouth under water. • Keep toilet lids down and bathroom doors closed.
Poisoning	• Keep house plants and cleaning agents out of reach. • Place poisons, paint, and gasoline in locked cabinets. • Keep medications in child-proof containers and locked up. • Dispose of medications that are no longer used or are out of date.
Falls	• Keep crib and playpen rails up. • Never leave the infant unattended on a changing table or other high surface. • Restrain when in high chair, swing, stroller, etc. • Place in a low bed when toddler starts to climb.
Motor vehicle/ Injury	• Use backward facing car seat until the infant/toddler is 1 year old and weighs at least 20 lb. • All car seats should be federally approved and be placed in the back seat.
Burns	• Test the temperature of formula and bath water. • Place pots on back burners and turn handles away from the front of stove. • Supervise use of faucets.

RISK	PREVENTION EDUCATION
Preschoolers and school-age children	
Drowning	• Be sure the child has learned to swim and knows rules of water safety. • Place locked fences around home and neighborhood pools.
Motor vehicle/ Injury	• Use booster seats for children who are less than 4 feet, 9 inches tall and weigh less than 40 lb. (Usually 4 to 8 years old). The child should be able to sit with his back against the car seat and his legs should dangle over the seat. • Use seat belts properly after booster seats are no longer necessary. • Ensure the use of protective equipment for sports or bike riding. • Supervise and teach safe use of equipment. • Teach the child to play in safe areas. • Teach the child safety rules of the road. • Teach the child what to do if approached by stranger. • Begin sex education for school-age children.
Burns	• Reduce setting on water heater to no higher than 120° F. • Teach dangers of playing with matches, fireworks, firearms. • Teach school-age children how to properly use microwave and other cooking instruments.
Poison	• Teach the child about the hazards of alcohol and prescription, non-prescription, and illegal drugs. • Keep potentially dangerous substances out of reach.
Adolescents	
Motor vehicle/ Injury	• Ensure the teen has completed a driver education course. • Set rules for the number of people allowed to ride in the car and for seat belt use • Tell the teen to call for a ride home if a driver is impaired. • Reinforce teaching on proper use of protective equipment when participating in sports. • Be alert to signs of depression. • Teach about the hazards of firearms and safety precautions with firearms. • Teach to check water depth before diving.
Burns	• Teach to use sun block and protective clothing. • Teach dangers of sun bathing and tanning beds. • Educate on the hazards of smoking.

- Safety Risks and Prevention Measures for Young and Middle Age Adults

  o Motor vehicle crashes are the most common cause of death and injury to the adult. Occupational injuries contribute to the injury and death rate of the adult. High consumption of alcohol and suicide are also major concerns for adults.

  o Nurses can promote client safety for young and middle age adults by:

    ▪ Reminding clients to drive defensively and to not drive after drinking alcohol

- Reinforcing teaching about the long-term effects related to high alcohol consumption

- Being attuned to behaviors that suggest the presence of depression and/or thoughts of suicide and referring clients as appropriate

- Encouraging clients to become proactive about safety in the work place

- Ensuring that clients understand the hazards of excessive sun exposure and the need to protect the skin with the use of sun-blocking agents and protective clothing

o Safety Risks and Prevention Measures for Older Adults

- The rate at which age-related changes occur varies greatly among older adults.

- Many older adults are able to maintain a lifestyle that promotes independence and the ability to protect themselves from safety hazards.

- Risk factors for injuries for older adults include:

  □ Physical, cognitive, and sensory changes

  □ Changes in the musculoskeletal and neurological systems (falls)

  □ Vision and/or hearing impairment (falls)

  □ Frequent trips to the bathroom at night because of nocturia and incontinence (falls)

  □ A decrease in tactile sensitivity (burns, other types of tissue injury)

- When the client demonstrates factors that increases the risk for injury (regardless of age), a home hazard evaluation should be conducted by a nurse, a physical therapist, and/or occupational therapist. The client is made aware of the environmental factors that may pose a risk to safety and suggested modifications.

- Modifications that can be made to improve home safety include:

  □ Removing items that could cause the client to trip, such as throw rugs and loose carpets

  □ Placing electrical cords and extension cords against a wall behind furniture

  □ Making sure that steps and sidewalks are in good repair

  □ Placing grab bars near the toilet and in the tub or shower and installing a stool riser

  □ Using a non-skid mat in the tub or shower

  □ Placing a shower chair in the shower

  □ Ensuring that lighting is adequate both inside and outside of the home

NURSING LEADERSHIP AND MANAGEMENT

Fire Safety in the Home

- Home fires continue to be a major cause of death and injury for people of all ages.

- It is imperative that nurses educate clients about the importance of developing a home safety plan that includes the following:

  o Keep emergency numbers near the phone for prompt use in the event of an emergency of any type.

  o Ensure that the number and placement of fire extinguishers and smoke alarms are adequate and that they are operable. Set a specific time to routinely change the batteries in the smoke alarms (in the fall when the clocks are set back to standard time and spring when reset at daylight savings time).

  o Have a family exit and meeting plan for fires that is reviewed and practiced regularly. Be sure to include closing windows and doors if able and to exit a smoke filled area by covering the mouth and nose with a damp cloth and getting down as close to the floor as possible.

  o Review with clients of all ages that in the event that the client's clothing or skin is on fire the mnemonic "Stop, Drop, and Roll" should be used to extinguish the fire.

  o If oxygen is being used in the home, oxygen safety measures should be reviewed. Because oxygen can cause materials to combust more easily and burn more rapidly, the client and family must be provided with information on use of the oxygen delivery equipment and the dangers of combustion. The following information should be included in the teaching plan:

    ▪ Use and store oxygen equipment according to the manufacturer's recommendations.

    ▪ Place a NO SMOKING sign in a conspicuous place near the front door of the home. A sign may also be placed on the door to the client's bedroom.

    ▪ Inform the client and family of the danger of smoking in the presence of oxygen. Family members and visitors who smoke should do so outside the home.

    ▪ Ensure that electrical equipment is in good repair and well grounded.

    ▪ Replace bedding that can generate static electricity (wool, nylon, synthetics) with items made from cotton.

    ▪ Keep flammable materials, such as heating oil and nail polish remover, away from the client when oxygen is in use.

    ▪ Follow general measures for fire safety in the home, such as having a fire extinguisher readily available and an established exit route should a fire occur.

Additional Risks in the Home and Community

- Additional risks in the home and community include passive smoking, carbon monoxide poisoning, and food poisoning. Bioterrorism has also become a concern, making disaster plans a mandatory part of community safety.

- Nurses should teach clients about the dangers of these additional risks.

  - Passive Smoking

    - Passive smoking is the unintentional inhalation of tobacco smoke.

    - Exposure to nicotine and other toxins places people at risk for numerous diseases, including cancer, heart disease, and lung infections.

    - Low birth weight, prematurity, stillbirths, and sudden infant death syndrome (SIDS) have been associated with maternal smoking.

    - Passive smoking is associated with childhood development of bronchitis, pneumonia, and middle ear infections.

    - For children with asthma, exposure to passive smoke can result in an increase in the frequency and the severity of asthma attacks.

    - Nurses should inform clients who smoke and their families about:

      - The hazards of smoking

      - Available resources to stop smoking (smoking cessation programs, medication support, self-help groups)

      - The effect that visiting individuals who smoke or riding in the automobile of a smoker has on a non-smoker

  - Carbon Monoxide

    - Carbon monoxide is a very dangerous gas because it binds with hemoglobin and ultimately reduces the oxygen supplied to tissues in the body.

    - Carbon monoxide cannot be seen, smelled, or tasted.

    - Symptoms of carbon monoxide poisoning include nausea, vomiting, headache, weakness, and unconsciousness.

    - Death may occur with prolonged exposure.

    - Measures to prevent carbon monoxide poisoning include ensuring proper ventilation when using fuel-burning devices (lawn mowers, wood burning and gas fireplaces, charcoal grills).

    - Gas burning furnaces, water heaters, and appliances should be inspected annually.

    - Flues and chimneys should be unobstructed.

    - Carbon monoxide detectors should be installed and inspected regularly.

- ○ Food Poisoning
  - ■ Food poisoning is a major cause of illness in the United States.
  - ■ Most food poisoning is caused by some type of bacteria, such as *Escherichia coli*, *Listeria monocytogenes*, and *Salmonella*.
  - ■ Healthy individuals usually recover from the illness in a few days.
  - ■ Very young, very old, pregnant women, and immunocompromised individuals are at risk for complications.
  - ■ Clients who are especially at risk are instructed to follow a low-microbial diet.
  - ■ Most food poisoning occurs because of unsanitary food practice.
  - ■ Proper hand hygiene, ensuring that meat and fish are cooked to the correct temperature, handling raw and fresh food separately to avoid cross contamination, and refrigerating perishable items are measures that may prevent food poisoning.
- ○ Bioterrorism
  - ■ Bioterrorism is the dissemination of harmful toxins, bacteria, viruses, or pathogens for the purpose of causing illness or death.
  - ■ Anthrax, variola, *Clostridium botulinum*, and *Yersinia pestis* are examples of types of agents used by terrorists.
  - ■ Nurses and other health professionals must be prepared to respond to an attack by being proficient in early detection, recognizing the causative agent, identifying the affected community, and providing early treatment to affected persons. For more information, go to the Web site of the Association of Professionals in Infection Control and Epidemiology (http://www.apic.org/).

ERGONOMIC PRINCIPLES

 Overview

- Ergonomics are the factors or qualities in an object's design and/or use that contribute to comfort, safety, efficiency, and ease of use.
- Body mechanics is the proper use of muscles to maintain balance, posture, and body alignment when performing a physical task. Nurses use body mechanics when providing care to clients by lifting, bending, and carrying out the activities of daily living.
- The risk of injury to the client and the nurse is reduced with the use of good body mechanics. Whenever possible, mechanical lift devices should be used to lift and transfer clients. Many health care agencies have "no manual lift" and "no solo lift" policies.

Safety Measures

- Guidelines to Prevent Injury

    o Know your agency's policies regarding lifting.

    o Plan ahead for activities that require lifting, transfer, or ambulation of a client and ask other staff members to be ready to assist at the time planned.

    o Be aware that the safest way to lift a client may be with the use of assistive equipment.

    o Rest between heavy lifting activities to decrease muscle fatigue.

    o Maintain good posture and exercise regularly to increase the strength of arm, leg, back, and abdominal muscles so these activities require less energy.

    o Use smooth movements when lifting and moving clients to prevent injury through sudden or jerky muscle movements.

    o When standing for long periods of time, flex the hip and knee through use of a foot rest. When sitting for long periods of time, keep the knees slightly higher than the hips.

    o Avoid repetitive movements of the hands, wrists, and shoulders. Take a break every 15 to 20 min to flex and stretch joints and muscles.

    o Maintain good posture (head and neck in straight line with pelvis) to avoid neck flexion and hunched shoulders, which can cause impingement of nerves in the neck.

    o Avoid twisting the spine or bending at the waist (flexion) to minimize the risk for injury.

- Center of Gravity

    o The center of gravity is the center of a mass.

    o Weight is a quantity of matter acted on by the force of gravity .

    o To lift an object, the nurse must overcome the weight of the object and know the center of gravity of the object.

    o When the human body is in the upright position, the center of gravity is the pelvis.

    o When an individual moves, the center of gravity shifts.

    o The closer the line of gravity is to the center of the base of support, the more stable the individual is.

    o To lower the center of gravity, bend the hips and knees.

- Lifting

    o Use the major muscle groups to prevent back strain, and tighten the abdominal muscles to increase support to the back muscles.

    o Distribute the weight between the large muscles of the arms and legs to decrease the strain on any one muscle group and avoid strain on smaller muscles.

NURSING LEADERSHIP AND MANAGEMENT

- When lifting an object from the floor, flex the hips, knees, and back. Get the object to thigh level keeping the knees bent and straightening the back. Stand up while holding the object as close as possible to the body, bringing the load to the center of gravity to increase stability and decrease back strain.

- Use assistive devices whenever possible and seek assistance whenever it is needed.

- Pushing or Pulling a Load

  - Widen the base of support.

  - When opportunity allows, pull objects toward the center of gravity rather than pushing away.

  - If pushing, move the front foot forward and, if pulling, move the rear leg back to promote stability.

  - Face the direction of movement when moving a client.

  - Use own body as a counter weight when pushing or pulling, which makes the movement easier.

  - Sliding, rolling, and pushing require less energy than lifting and have less risk for injury.

  - Avoid twisting the thoracic spine and bending the back while the hips and knees are straight.

- Transfers and Use of Assistive Devices

  - Assess the client's ability to help with transfers (balance, muscle strength, endurance).

  - Determine the need for additional personnel or assistive devices (transfer belt, hydraulic lift, sliding board).

  - Assess and monitor the client's use of mobility aids (canes, walkers, crutches).

  - Include assistance or mobility aids needed for safe transfers and ambulation in plan of care.

CHAPTER 4: MAINTAINING A SAFE ENVIRONMENT

 Application Exercises

1. A home health nurse is assessing the safety of a client's home. Which of the following factors may increase the client's risk for falls? (Select all that apply.)

    _____   History of a previous fall

    _____   Reduced vision

    _____   Impaired memory

    _____   Antibiotic therapy

    _____   House slippers

    _____   Kyphosis (hump back curvature of the spine)

2. A client is brought back to the unit after a total hip arthroplasty. The client is confused, is moving the operated leg into positions that could dislocate the new hip joint, and repeatedly attempts to get out of bed. Which of the following actions should the nurse take? (Select all that apply.)

    _____   Apply arm and leg restraints immediately.

    _____   Get an order from the primary care provider.

    _____   Have a family member sign the consent for the restraints.

    _____   Use a square knot to secure the restraints to the bed.

    _____   Document on the plan of care for neuro checks of the extremities to be done every 4 hr.

    _____   Ensure that only one finger can be inserted between the restraint and the client.

3. A nurse is observing a newly licensed nurse pull a client up in bed using a drawsheet with an assistive personnel (AP). Which of the following actions by the newly licensed nurse indicates a need for further education?

    A. The nurse spreads his legs apart.

    B. The nurse uses his body weight to counter the client's weight.

    C. The nurse's feet are facing inward, toward the center of the bed.

    D. The nurse uses the muscles in his arms to lift the client off the bed using the drawsheet.

4. An AP reports that a client's fingerstick blood glucose reading 30 min before lunch is 58 mg/dL. The client's morning fingerstick blood glucose was 285 mg/dL. The client is asymptomatic for hypoglycemia, and additional insulin is scheduled to be administered at this time. Which of the following actions should the nurse take first?

    A. Recalibrate the glucometer and recheck the client's blood glucose.

    B. Have the laboratory draw a stat serum glucose.

    C. Inform the AP to give the client 120 mL of orange juice.

    D. Administer insulin as prescribed.

5. A nurse in the ICU is assigned to a client with multisystem failure. The client is on cardiac monitoring and receiving mechanical ventilation. Wall suction is set up, an indwelling urinary catheter is draining by gravity, TPN is infusing, and antibiotics are being given intermittently through a central venous access device. In addition, 2 units of packed RBCs have been prescribed. What actions should the nurse take to ensure all equipment is properly working and the client is in a safe environment?

CHAPTER 4: MAINTAINING A SAFE ENVIRONMENT

 Application Exercises Answer Key

1. A home health nurse is assessing the safety of a client's home. Which of the following factors may increase the client's risk for falls? (Select all that apply.)

__X__	**History of a previous fall**
__X__	**Reduced vision**
__X__	**Impaired memory**
_____	Antibiotic therapy
__X__	**House slippers**
__X__	**Kyphosis (hump back curvature of the spine)**

All of the above factors except antibiotic therapy can increase a client's risk for falls. A history of falls is a significant risk factor; reduced vision may make it difficult for the client to avoid mishaps with equipment and furniture in the environment; clients with impaired memory may find it difficult to remember to ask for help with ambulation and ADLs; house slippers may not provide adequate traction and support for safe ambulation; and kyphosis alters an individual's posture and center of balance.

 NCLEX® Connection: Safety and Infection Control, Home Safety

2. A client is brought back to the unit after a total hip arthroplasty. The client is confused, is moving the operated leg into positions that could dislocate the new hip joint, and repeatedly attempts to get out of bed. Which of the following actions should the nurse take? (Select all that apply.)

__X__	**Apply arm and leg restraints immediately.**
__X__	**Get an order from the primary care provider.**
__X__	**Have a family member sign the consent for the restraints.**
_____	Use a square knot to secure the restraints to the bed.
_____	Document on the plan of care for neuro checks of the extremities to be done every 4 hr.
_____	Ensure that only one finger can be inserted between the restraint and the client.

In a situation where the client is in imminent danger of doing harm to himself, the nurse may apply restraints prior to notifying the provider. The provider does need to be notified immediately for a prescription for restraints, and a family member must sign a consent for the restraints. A quick release knot should be used to secure the restraint to the bed; neuro checks of the extremities should be done at least every 2 hr; and two finger widths should be the distance between the restraint and the client.

 NCLEX® Connection: Safety and Infection Control, Injury Prevention

NURSING LEADERSHIP AND MANAGEMENT

3. A nurse is observing a newly licensed nurse pull a client up in bed using a drawsheet with an assistive personnel (AP). Which of the following actions by the newly licensed nurse indicates a need for further education?

    A. The nurse spreads his legs apart.

    B. The nurse uses his body weight to counter the client's weight.

    C. The nurse's feet are facing inward, toward the center of the bed.

    D. The nurse uses the muscles in his arms to lift the client off the bed using the drawsheet.

The nurse should face the direction of movement when moving a client. Subsequently, the nurse's feet should be pointing at the head of the bed instead of the center of the bed. All the other actions are correct.

 NCLEX® Connection: Safety and Infection Control, Injury Prevention

4. An AP reports that a client's fingerstick blood glucose reading 30 min before lunch is 58 mg/dL. The client's morning fingerstick blood glucose was 285 mg/dL. The client is asymptomatic for hypoglycemia, and additional insulin is scheduled to be administered at this time. Which of the following actions should the nurse take first?

    A. Recalibrate the glucometer and recheck the client's blood glucose.

    B. Have the laboratory draw a stat serum glucose.

    C. Inform the AP to give the client 120 mL of orange juice.

    D. Administer insulin as prescribed.

Since the client's blood glucose was high in the morning and is now so low, the blood glucose should be rechecked after recalibrating the glucometer to ensure the reading was accurate before any interventions are taken.

 NCLEX® Connection: Safety and Infection Control, Safe Use of Equipment

5. A nurse in the ICU is assigned to a client with multisystem failure. The client is on cardiac monitoring and receiving mechanical ventilation. Wall suction is set up, an indwelling urinary catheter is draining by gravity, TPN is infusing, and antibiotics are being given intermittently through a central venous access device. In addition, 2 units of packed RBCs have been prescribed. What actions should the nurse take to ensure all equipment is properly working and the client is in a safe environment?

The nurse should check that: The ventilator is plugged in to an outlet that is designated to be powered by a backup generator; all machines hooked to electricity have ground plugs and are plugged directly into wall sockets; wall suction is set at the proper settings for suction; the ventilator is properly set according to the provider's prescriptions; the indwelling urinary catheter is not kinked and is properly taped to the client to avoid damage to the bladder or urethra; IV pumps have free-flow protection devices; lumens of the catheter are clamped and, if not in use, properly capped; 0.9% sodium chloride is available for administration of packed cells; the blood pressure cuff is properly applied; pulse oximetry is properly applied and giving accurate readings; a sterile dressing kit is available for care of the central line; and ECG leads are intact and properly placed with good capture of rhythm.

 NCLEX® Connection: Safety and Infection Control, Safe Use of Equipment

CHAPTER 5: FACILITY PROTOCOLS

- Reporting Incidents
- Disaster Planning and Emergency Response
- Security Plans

NCLEX® CONNECTIONS

When reviewing the content in this chapter, keep in mind the relevant sections of the NCLEX® outline, in particular:

CLIENT NEEDS: SAFETY AND INFECTION CONTROL

Relevant topics/tasks include:
- Emergency Response Plan
  - Use clinical decision-making/critical thinking for emergency response plan.
- Reporting of Incident/Event/Irregular Occurrence/Variance
  - Evaluate response to error/event/occurrence.
- Security Plan
  - Use clinical decision making/critical thinking in situations related to security planning.

Chapter 5	Facility Protocols

 Overview

- Facility protocols refer to the plans and procedures in place to address specific issues that health care institutions face.

- Nurses must understand their role in relation to the development and implementation of facility protocols, which include:

  o Reporting Incidents

  o Disaster Planning and Emergency Response

  o Security Plans

REPORTING INCIDENTS

 Overview

- Incident reports are records made of unexpected or unusual incidents that affected a client, volunteer, or visitor in a health care facility.

- Incident reports may also be referred to as "unusual occurrence reports" by an institution.

- In most states, incident reports cannot be subpoenaed by clients or used as evidence in lawsuits.

- Incidents that require a report include but are not limited to:

  o Medication errors

  o Procedure/treatment errors

  o Equipment-related injuries/errors

  o Needlestick injuries

  o Client falls/injuries

  o Visitor/volunteer injuries

  o Threat made to client or staff

  o Loss of property (dentures, wedding ring, personal wheelchair)

    ▪ Nurses must ensure the safety of clients' valuables. If a client is admitted to the emergency department and is not accompanied by a family member, the client's personal items should be placed in an envelope and given to security. If an individual claims to be a family member, the client must identify the person and give that person permission to be in possession of the valuables.

Nursing Role in Reporting Incidents

- In the event of an incident that involves a client, volunteer, or visitor, the nurse's first responsibility is to assess the individual for injuries and institute any immediate care measures necessary to decrease further injury. If it was a client-related incident, the provider should then be notified, and additional tests or treatment should be carried out as prescribed.

- Nurses should recognize that incident reports:

    o Should be completed by the person who identifies that an unexpected event has occurred (this may or may not be the individual most directly involved in the incident).

    o Should be completed as soon as possible and within 24 hr of the incident.

    o Are considered confidential and are not shared with the client (nor is it acknowledged to the client that one was completed).

    o Are not placed in the client's chart nor mentioned in the client's medical record; however, a description of the incident itself should be documented factually in the client's record.

    o Include an objective description of the incident and actions taken to safeguard the client, as well as assessment and treatment of any injuries sustained.

    o Are forwarded to the risk management department or officer (varies from facility to facility), possibly after being reviewed by the nurse manager.

    o Provide data that may be used in performance improvement studies regarding the incidence of client injuries and care-related errors.

- The incident report itself should include:

    o The client's name and hospital number (or visitor's name and address if visitor injury), along with the date, time, and location of the incident

    o A factual description of the incident and injuries incurred, avoiding any assumptions as to the cause of the incident

    o Names of any witnesses to the incident and any client or witness comments regarding the incident

    o Corrective actions that were taken, including notification of the provider and any referrals

    o The name and dose of any medication or identification number of any piece of equipment that was involved in the incident

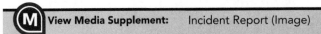

View Media Supplement: Incident Report (Image)

DISASTER PLANNING AND EMERGENCY RESPONSE

 Overview

- A disaster is a mass casualty or intrafacility event that overwhelms or interrupts, at least temporarily, the normal flow of services of a hospital.

- Disasters that health care facilities face include internal and external emergencies.

  ○ Internal emergencies are events that occur within a facility and include loss of electric power or potable water and severe damage or casualties related to fire, severe weather (tornado, hurricane), an explosion, or a terrorist act. Internal emergency readiness includes safety and hazardous materials protocols and infection control policies and practices.

  ○ External emergencies are events that affect a facility indirectly and include severe weather (tornado, hurricane), volcanic eruptions, earthquakes, pandemic flu, chemical plant explosions, industrial accidents, building collapses, major transportation accidents, and terrorist acts (including biological and chemical warfare). External emergency readiness includes a plan for participation in community-wide emergencies and disasters.

- Nurses should be aware that all health care facilities have color code designations for emergencies. These may vary between institutions but some examples are:

  - Code Red (fire)
  - Code Pink (newborn abduction)
  - Code Orange (chemical spill)
  - Code Blue (mass casualty incident)
  - Code Gray (tornado)

- Nurses should be familiar with procedures and policies that outline proper measures to take when one of these emergencies are called.

The Joint Commission and Emergency Preparedness

- The Joint Commission (www.jointcommission.org) has established emergency preparedness management standards for various types of health care facilities. These standards mandate that an institutional emergency preparedness plan be developed by all health care institutions and that these plans include institution-specific procedures for:

  ○ Notifying personnel and assigning responsibilities

  ○ Notifying external authorities of emergencies

  ○ Managing space and supplies and providing security

  ○ Radioactive or chemical isolation and decontamination (measures to contain contamination, decontamination at scene of exposure)

- Evacuation and setting up an alternative care site when the facility cannot support adequate client care and treatment
    - Critical processes when an alternative care site is necessary include:
        - Client information/care packaging (admissions, medical records, medications, and tracking of transfers)
        - Interfacility communication
        - Transportation of clients, staff, and equipment
        - Cross-privileging of medical staff
- Triage of incoming clients
- Management of clients during emergencies, including scheduling, modification or discontinuation of services, control of client information, and client discharge and transportation
- Interaction with family members and the news media
- Identification of backup resources (electricity, water, fire protection, fuel sources, medical gas and vacuum) for utilities and communication
- Orientation and education of personnel who will participate in implementation of the emergency preparedness plan
- Crisis support for health care workers (access to vaccines, infection control advice, mental health counseling)
- Performance monitoring and evaluation related to emergency preparedness.
- Conducting two emergency preparedness drills each year
    - Drills should include an influx of clients beyond those being treated by the facility.
    - Drills should include either an internal or an external disaster (a situation beyond the normal capacity of the facility).

Nursing Role in Disaster Planning and Emergency Response

- Emergency Response Plans
    - Each health care institution must have an emergency preparedness plan that has been developed by a planning committee. This committee reviews information regarding the potential for various types of natural and man-made emergencies depending on the characteristics of the community. Resources necessary to meet the potential emergency are also determined, and a plan is developed that takes into consideration all of these factors.
    - Nurses, as well as a cross section of other members of the health care team, should be involved in the development of an emergency operations plan (EOP) for such emergencies. Criteria under which the EOP are activated should be clear. Roles for each employee should be outlined and administrative control determined. A designated area for the area command center should be established, as well as a person to serve as the incident control manager.

NURSING LEADERSHIP AND MANAGEMENT

- Triage

  o Principles of triage should be followed in health care institutions involved in a mass casualty event.

  o These differ from the principles of triage that are typically followed during provision of day-to-day services in an emergency or urgent care setting. During mass casualty events, casualties are separated in relation to their potential for survival, and treatment is allocated accordingly.

  o Categories of triage during mass casualty events

    ▪ Emergent category (class I) – Highest priority is given to clients who have life-threatening injuries but also have a high possibility of survival once they are stabilized.

    ▪ Urgent category (class II) – Second highest priority is given to clients who have major injuries that are not yet life threatening and can usually wait 45 to 60 min for treatment.

    ▪ Nonurgent category (class III) – The next highest priority is given to clients who have minor injuries that are not life threatening and do not need immediate attention.

    ▪ Expectant category (class IV) – The lowest priority is given to clients who are not expected to live and will be allowed to die naturally. Comfort measures may be provided, but restorative care will not.

- Discharge/Relocation of Clients

  o During an emergency such as a fire or a mass casualty event, decisions may need to be made regarding discharging clients or relocating them so their bed can be given to clients with higher priority needs.

  o Criteria should be followed when identifying clients who can be safely discharged.

    ▪ Ambulatory clients requiring minimal care should be discharged or relocated first.

    ▪ Clients requiring assistance should be next and arrangements should made for continuation of their care.

    ▪ Clients who are unstable and/or require nursing care should not be discharged or relocated unless they are in imminent danger.

- Fire

  o If a nurse discovers a fire that threatens the safety of a client, the nurse should use the RACE mnemonic (Rescue, Alarm, Contain, Extinguish) to guide the order of actions.

RACE MNEMONIC	
Rescue	• Rescue the client and other individuals from the area.
Alarm	• Pull the fire alarm, which will activate the EMS response system. • Systems that could increase fire spread are automatically shut down with activation of the alarm.
Contain	• Once the room or area has been cleared, the door leading to the area in which the fire is located as well as the fire doors should be kept closed in order to contain the fire. • Fire doors should be kept closed as much as possible when moving from area to area within the facility to avoid the spread of smoke and fire.
Extinguish	• Make an attempt to extinguish small fires by using a single fire extinguisher, smothering it with a blanket, or dousing it with water (except with an electrical or grease fire). • Complete evacuation of the area should occur if the nurse cannot put the fire out with these methods. • Attempts at extinguishing the fire should only be made when the employee has been properly trained in the safe and proper use of a fire extinguisher and when only one extinguisher is needed.

- Severe Thunderstorm/Tornado

  o Draw all shades and close all drapes to protect against shattering glass.

  o Lower all beds to the lowest position and move beds away from the windows.

  o Place blankets over all clients who are confined to beds.

  o Close all doors.

  o Get as many ambulatory clients as possible into the hallways (away from windows).

  o Do not use elevators.

  o Turn on the severe weather channel to monitor severe weather warnings.

- Biological Incidents

  o Take measures to protect self and others.

  o Recognize signs and symptoms of infection/poisoning and implement appropriate treatment.

INCIDENT	SIGNS AND SYMPTOMS	TREATMENT/PREVENTION
Inhalational anthrax	<ul><li>Sore throat</li><li>Fever</li><li>Muscle aches</li><li>Severe dyspnea</li><li>Meningitis</li><li>Shock</li></ul>	<ul><li>IV ciprofloxacin (Cipro)</li></ul>
Botulism	<ul><li>Difficulty swallowing</li><li>Progressive weakness</li><li>Nausea, vomiting, abdominal cramps</li><li>Difficulty breathing</li></ul>	<ul><li>Airway management</li><li>Antitoxin</li><li>Elimination of toxin</li></ul>
Smallpox	<ul><li>High fever</li><li>Fatigue</li><li>Severe headache</li><li>Rash (starts centrally and spreads outward) that turns to pus-filled lesions</li><li>Vomiting</li><li>Delirium</li><li>Excessive bleeding</li></ul>	<ul><li>Treatment: No cure</li><li>Supportive care: Hydration, pain medication, antipyretics</li><li>Prevention: Vaccine</li></ul>
Ebola	<ul><li>Sore throat</li><li>Headache</li><li>High temperature</li><li>Nausea, vomiting, diarrhea</li><li>Internal and external bleeding</li><li>Shock</li></ul>	<ul><li>Treatment: No cure</li><li>Supportive care: Minimize invasive procedures</li><li>Prevention: Vaccine</li></ul>

- Chemical Incidents

  o Take measures to protect self and to avoid contact.

  o Assess and intervene to maintain the client's airway, breathing, and circulation and administer first aid as needed.

  o Effectively remove the offending chemical by undressing the client and removing all identifiable particulate matter. Decontaminate the client by providing immediate and prolonged irrigations of contaminated areas.

  o Gather a specific history of the injury, if possible (name and concentration of the chemical, duration of exposure).

  o In the event of a chemical attack, have knowledge of which facilities are open to exposed clients and which are only open to unexposed clients.

  o Follow the facility's emergency response plans (personal protection measures, handling and disposal of wastes, use of space and equipment, reporting).

- Hazardous Material Incidents

  o Take measures to protect self and to avoid contact.

  o Approach the scene with caution.

  o Attempt to identify the hazardous material with available resources (emergency response guidebook, poison control centers). Have knowledge of where the Material Safety Data Sheets (MSDS) manual is located.

  o Try to contain the material in one place prior to the arrival of the hazardous materials team.

  o If individuals are contaminated, decontaminate them as much as possible at the scene or as close as possible to the scene.

    ▪ With few exceptions, water is the universal antidote. For biological hazardous materials, wash skin with copious amounts of water and antibacterial soap.

    ▪ Don gloves, a gown, a mask, and shoe covers to protect self from contamination.

    ▪ Carefully and slowly remove contaminated clothing so that deposited material does not become airborne.

    ▪ Put contaminated materials into large plastic bags and seal them.

- Radiological Incidents

  o The amount of exposure is related to the duration of exposure, distance from source, and amount of shielding.

  o The facility in which victims are cared for should activate interventions to prevent exposure of treatment areas (floors and furniture should be covered, air vents and ducts should be covered, radiation-contaminated waste should be disposed according to procedural guidelines).

  o Staff should wear water-resistant gowns, double glove, and fully cover their bodies with caps, booties, masks, and goggles.

  o Staff should wear radiation or dosimetry badges to monitor the amount of their radiation exposure.

  o Clients should initially be surveyed with a radiation meter to determine amount of contamination.

  o Decontamination with soap and water and disposable towels should occur prior to the client entering the hospital. Water runoff will be contaminated and should be contained.

  o After decontamination, clients should be resurveyed for residual contamination, and washing should be continued until the client is clean of all contamination.

- Bomb Threat

  o When a phone call is received:

    ▪ Extend the conversation as long as possible.

    ▪ Listen for distinguishing background noises (music, voices, traffic, airplanes).

- ■ Note any distinguishing voice characteristics of the caller.

- ■ Ask where and at what time the bomb is set to explode.

- ■ Note if the caller is familiar with the physical arrangement of the facility.

- ○ If a bomb-like device is located, do not touch it. Clear the area and isolate the device as much as possible by, for example, closing doors.

- ○ Notify the appropriate authorities and personnel (police, administrator, director of nursing).

- ○ Cooperate with police and others – assist to conduct search as needed, provide copies of floor plans, have master keys available, and watch for and isolate suspicious objects such as packages and boxes.

- ○ Keep elevators available for authorities.

- ○ Remain calm and alert and try not to alarm clients.

SECURITY PLANS

 Overview

- • All health care facilities should have security plans in place that include preventive, protective, and response measures designed for identified security needs.

- • Security issues faced by health care facilities include: admission of potentially dangerous individuals, vandalism, infant abduction, and information theft.

- • The International Association for Healthcare Security & Safety (IAHSS) provides recommendations for the development of security plans.

Nursing Role in Security Plans

- • Nurses should be aware that security measures include:

  - ■ An identification system that identifies employees, volunteers, physicians, students, and regularly scheduled contract services staff as authorized personnel of the health care facility

  - ■ Electronic security systems in high-risk areas (the newborn nursery to prevent infant abductions, the emergency department to prevent unauthorized entrance)

    - □ Key code access into and out of newborn nurseries

    - □ Wrist bands that electronically link the mother and her infant

    - □ Alarms integrated with closed-circuit television cameras

- • Nurses should be prepared to take immediate action when breaches in security occur. Time is of the essence in stopping an abduction or the theft of confidential information.

CHAPTER 5: FACILITY PROTOCOLS

 Application Exercises

1. A nurse realizes that a client was administered an antihypertensive medication intended for another client. Number the following actions in the appropriate sequence that the nurse should follow.

_____ Call the client's primary care provider.

_____ Take the client's vital signs.

_____ Notify the risk management officer.

_____ Complete an incident report.

_____ Instruct the client to remain in bed until further notice.

2. Which of the following statements are true of incident reports? (Select all that apply.)

_____ A description of the incident should be documented in the nursing notes.

_____ Incident reports are confidential and should not be shared with the client.

_____ Incident reports include a description of the incident and actions taken.

_____ A copy of the incident report should be placed in the client's chart.

_____ The risk management department investigates the incident.

3. An individual approaches the door of the newborn nursery and claims that he is the father of an infant. He is unable to provide the infant's code that was provided to the family. Which of the following actions should the nurse take?

   A. Ask the man several discriminating questions, such as the mother's name and time of birth, and admit him if he can answer them.

   B. Call security to remove the man from the area.

   C. Ask the man to obtain the infant's code from the mother and then return.

   D. Call a Code Pink, since the man could be attempting to abduct the infant.

4. A community experiences an outbreak of meningitis, and hospital beds are urgently needed. Which of the following clients is appropriate to discharge?

   A. 58-year-old man admitted this morning with angina and a history of a CABG 1 year ago

   B. 50-year-old adult with type 2 diabetes mellitus being admitted for rotator cuff surgery

   C. 70-year-old adult admitted yesterday with pneumonia and dehydration

   D. 65-year-old woman who fell and broke her hip and is scheduled for total hip replacement tomorrow

5. Which of the following nursing actions are appropriate if a severe weather alarm is activated? (Select all that apply.)

_____ Draw shades and close drapes as protection against shattering glass.

_____ Lower beds to the lowest position and move beds away from the windows as much as possible.

_____ Keep doors open to facilitate quick evacuation of clients.

_____ Get as many ambulatory clients as possible into the hallways.

_____ Use the elevators to move clients to lower levels.

_____ Turn the radio on for severe weather warnings.

6. A nurse enters a client's room and finds that a fire has started. Number the following actions in the appropriate sequence that the nurse should follow.

_____ Shut the fire doors on the unit.

_____ Move the client away from the fire.

_____ Activate the fire alarm.

_____ Extinguish the fire (if trained in using a fire extinguisher).

CHAPTER 5: FACILITY PROTOCOLS

 Application Exercises Answer Key

1. A nurse realizes that a client was administered an antihypertensive medication intended for another client. Number the following actions in the appropriate sequence that the nurse should follow.

__3__ Call the client's primary care provider.

__1__ Take the client's vital signs.

__5__ Notify the risk management officer.

__4__ Complete an incident report.

__2__ Instruct the client to remain in bed until further notice.

Since the medication administered can decrease blood pressure, the nurse should take the client's vital signs and instruct the client to remain in bed until the medication's effects can be assessed. The provider should then be notified of the error. The provider then may order a medication to counteract the antihypertensive's effects if the client's vital signs indicate this is necessary. The nurse must then complete an incident report and notify the risk management officer for proper disposition.

 NCLEX® Connection: Safety and Infection Control, Reporting of Incident/Event/Irregular Occurrence/Variance

2. Which of the following statements are true of incident reports? (Select all that apply.)

__X__ **A description of the incident should be documented in the nursing notes.**

__X__ **Incident reports are confidential and should not be shared with the client.**

__X__ **Incident reports include a description of the incident and actions taken.**

_____ A copy of the incident report should be placed in the client's chart.

__X__ **The risk management department investigates the incident.**

An incident report is confidential and not shared with the client. An incident report should include a description of the incident and actions taken to safeguard the client and/or assess and treat the injuries sustained. A risk management department usually investigates the incident. A copy of the incident report should not be placed in the client's chart, nor should a note be put in the chart that one was filled out. However, documentation of the incident should be recorded in the client's chart in regard to disposition of client, first aid administered, and any injuries that were incurred.

 NCLEX® Connection: Safety and Infection Control, Reporting of Incident/Event/Irregular Occurrence/Variance

3. An individual approaches the door of the newborn nursery and claims that he is the father of an infant. He is unable to provide the infant's code that was provided to the infant's family. Which of the following actions should the nurse take?

> A. Ask the man several discriminating questions, such as the mother's name and time of birth, and admit him if he can answer them.
>
> B. Call security to remove the man from the area.
>
> **C. Ask the man to obtain the infant's code from the mother and then return.**
>
> D. Call a Code Pink, since the man could be attempting to abduct the infant.

> **The nurse should initially ask the man to obtain the proper code from the infant's mother. If he returns with the code, he should be admitted. While asking the man discriminating questions may verify that he is the father, it does not follow the safety procedures outlined by the facility. It is premature to involve security or call a Code Pink, since the man has not made any threatening gestures that would warrant these actions.**

 NCLEX® Connection: Safety and Infection Control, Security Plan

4. A community experiences an outbreak of meningitis, and hospital beds are urgently needed. Which of the following clients is appropriate to discharge?

> A. 58-year-old man admitted this morning with angina and a history of a CABG 1 year ago
>
> **B. 50-year-old adult with type 2 diabetes mellitus being admitted for rotator cuff surgery**
>
> C. 70-year-old adult admitted yesterday with pneumonia and dehydration
>
> D. 65-year-old woman who fell and broke her hip and is scheduled for total hip replacement tomorrow

> **The client with type 2 diabetes mellitus is the most stable, and the surgery is not urgent. This client should be discharged and readmitted for surgery at a later date. The other three clients are experiencing acute disorders and should remain in the hospital.**

 NCLEX® Connection: Safety and Infection Control, Disaster Planning

5. Which of the following nursing actions are appropriate if a severe weather alarm is activated? (Select all that apply.)

    X   **Draw shades and close drapes as protection against shattering glass.**

    X   **Lower beds to the lowest position and move beds away from the windows as much as possible.**

           Keep doors open to facilitate quick evacuation of clients.

    X   **Get as many ambulatory clients as possible into the hallways.**

           Use the elevators to move clients to lower levels.

    X   **Turn the radio on for severe weather warnings.**

Measures such as drawing the shades, closing drapes, moving beds away from the window, and moving ambulatory clients into the hallway to protect them from shattering glass are appropriate. Doors should be kept closed and elevator use should be avoided.

 NCLEX® Connection: Safety and Infection Control, Disaster Planning

6. A nurse enters a client's room and finds that a fire has started. Number the following actions in the appropriate sequence that the nurse should follow.

    3   Shut the fire doors on the unit.

    1   Move the client away from the fire.

    2   Activate the fire alarm.

    4   Extinguish the fire (if trained in using a fire extinguisher).

Use the RACE mnemonic: rescue, alarm, contain, and extinguish.

Remove everyone from the area.

Pull the fire alarm, which will activate the EMS response.

Once the room or area has been cleared, the fire doors should be kept closed in order to contain the fire.

An attempt to extinguish the fire using a single fire extinguisher can be made only when practical and only when the employee has been properly trained in the safe and proper use of a fire extinguisher.

 NCLEX® Connection: Safety and Infection Control, Emergency Response Plan

References

Cherry, B., & Jacob, S. R. (2008). Contemporary nursing: Issues, trends, & management. (4th ed.). St. Louis, MO: Mosby, Inc.

Marquis, B.L., & Huston, C. J. (2009). Leadership roles and management functions in nursing: Theory and application. (6th ed.). Philadelphia: Lippincott Williams & Wilkins.

Nies, M., & McEwen, M. (2007). Community/public health nursing: Concepts of care in evidence-based practice. St. Louis, MO: Saunders.

Potter, P. A., & Perry, A. G. (2009). Fundamentals of nursing (7th ed.). St. Louis, MO: Mosby Elsevier.

Stanhope, M., & Lancaster, J. (2006). Foundations of nursing in the community (2nd ed.). St. Louis, MO: Mosby.

Varcarolis, E. M., Carson, V. B., & Shoemaker, N. C. (2006). Foundations of psychiatric mental health nursing: A clinical approach (5th ed.). St. Louis, MO: Saunders Elsevier.

Whitehead, D.K., Weiss, S. A., & Tappen, R. M. (2007). Essentials of nursing leadership and management. (4th ed.). Philadelphia: F.A. Davis Company.